CYSTIC FIBROSIS

MANUAL
DIAGNOSIS AND
MANAGEMENT

To

Thomas, Graeme and Alexander

All royalties from this book will be given to the
Cystic Fibrosis Research Trust
Alexandra House
5 Blyth Road, Bromley
Kent BR1 3RS

CYSTIC FIBROSIS

MANUAL OF DIAGNOSIS
AND MANAGEMENT

PREPARED BY

MARY C GOODCHILD
MD (B'ham), MB BS(Lond), DCH
Associate Specialist,
University Hospital of Wales, Cardiff

AND

JOHN A DODGE
MD (Wales), FRCP (Lond & Edin), DCH
Professor of Child Health,
Queen's University, Belfast, N Ireland
(formerly Reader in Child Health, University of Wales)

FOR

THE CYSTIC FIBROSIS
RESEARCH TRUST

SECOND EDITION

Baillière Tindall
LONDON PHILADELPHIA TORONTO
MEXICO CITY RIO DE JANEIRO SYDNEY TOKYO HONG KONG

<u>Baillière Tindall</u> 1 St Anne's Road
W. B. Saunders   Eastbourne, East Sussex BN21 3UN, England

West Washington Square
Philadelphia, PA 19105, USA

1 Goldthorne Avenue
Toronto, Ontario M8Z 5T9, Canada

Apartado 26370–Cedro 512
Mexico 4, DF Mexico

Rua Evaristo da Veiga 55, 10° andar
Rio de Janeiro–RJ, Brazil

ABP Australia Ltd, 44–50 Waterloo Road
North Ryde, NSW 2113, Australia

Ichibancho Central Building, 22- 1 Ichibancho
Chiyoda-ku, Tokyo 102, Japan

10/fl. Inter-Continental Plaza, 94 Granville Road
Tsim Sha Tsui East, Kowloon, Hong Kong

First published 1985

Printed and bound in Great Britain by
Biddles Ltd of Guildford, Surrey

British Library Cataloguing in Publication Data

Goodchild, Mary C.
   Cystic fibrosis: manual of diagnosis and
   management.—2nd ed.—
   1.Cystic fibrosis
   I.Title II.Dodge, John A. III. Anderson,
   Charlotte M. IV.Cystic Fibrosis Research Trust
   616.3'7   RC858.C95

ISBN 0-7020-1129-0

CONTENTS

PREFACE

Preparation of this manual was encouraged by the Medical and Scientific Advisory Committee of the Cystic Fibrosis Research Trust in the hope that it would supply the needs of those doctors and members of many other disciplines who approach the Trust for further information about cystic fibrosis.

The first edition, published in 1976, was written by Professor Charlotte M Anderson and Dr Mary C Goodchild. Professor Anderson, who directed cystic fibrosis clinics in Melbourne (Australia) and Birmingham (United Kingdom) for many years, has subsequently retired and relinquished co-authorship; the present authors record their gratitude to her for stimulation and advice.

During the nine years since the publication of the first edition, many advances have taken place, both in clinical management and research. Substantial rewriting has been required, therefore, in this second edition with an inevitable increase in size, but the format is similar to that of the original. References are not always specifically indicated throughout the text, but are given at the end of chapters, together with a mention of reviews or chapters from other books. An appendix describes the aims and activities of the Cystic Fibrosis Research Trust in the United Kingdom and lists publications. It also gives addresses of other CF organizations worldwide.

Both authors have been the grateful recipients of research grants from the Trust over a number of years. We should like to pay tribute to all those CF patients and their families who have taken part in research projects and who continue to raise money so generously and effectively for research funds.

We are indebted to many colleagues in the departments of Dietetics, Medical Illustration, Medical Microbiology, Pharmacy, Physiotherapy, Radiology and Social Work at the Children's Hospital, Birmingham and at the University Hospital of Wales, Cardiff. In particular, we should like to thank Mrs Anne Davies (Staff Pharmacist), Dr Margaret A McPherson and Dr H C Ryley (Biochemists), all at the University Hospital of Wales and Dr I A Campbell, Consultant Physician, Llandough Hospital, for their help with the relevant sections of the book.

We thank Mrs Betty Dickens of Baillière Tindall for her patience and support and we are especially grateful to Mrs Elizabeth Campbell for typing the manuscript, in its many versions, with skill and good humour.

Mary C Goodchild
John A Dodge

Chapter 1

THE NATURE OF CYSTIC FIBROSIS

INTRODUCTION

Cystic fibrosis of the pancreas, now known simply as *cystic fibrosis* or CF, has been recognized as a disease entity only since the late 1930s. It is the most common inherited disorder and the most frequent cause of chronic suppurative lung disease in children and young adults of Caucasian descent.

Until the early 1950s expectation of life, except in rare instances, was very short. Since then more effective treatment and perhaps earlier diagnosis, have led to a considerable improvement: a high proportion of children are now surviving to reach young adult life in good or at least in reasonable health and many are working members of the adult community. Although much is known about the clinical pattern and natural history of CF, its basic biochemical cause is still obscure. Treatment is aimed at the consequences and is still not curative. As these consequences are widespread throughout the body and tend to be progressive, treatment is complex and must be continued throughout life. In order to appreciate the importance of these many facets of management, a comprehensive understanding of the underlying pathophysiology is important.

The natural history of the condition is very variable. The clinical course in some will be better than in others, despite little or no treatment, or even with 'optimal' treatment. Nevertheless, the greater longevity in recent years must be due largely to the pattern of management which has been developed. At first the effectiveness of treatment was considered in terms of survival, but longevity alone is of dubious value without adequate well-being and the capacity to participate in a reasonably normal adult life: this is now the goal of 'optimal' management. Therefore when management is embarked upon early in life, it should be continued consistently, with some modifications at times, throughout life. A thorough and up-to-date knowledge of the treatment available and its value will be required by medical practitioners and other people dealing with these patients. **'Optimal' treatment, although it has its disappointments, can be extremely rewarding; suboptimal treatment may do little more than prolong the patient's life, without regard to the quality of that life.**

In this small book we aim to give an understanding of the many facets of the pathophysiology of cystic fibrosis and its management, not only to doctors but to a wide variety of paramedical personnel who will become involved in the varied treatment. It may be of use also to teachers and employers who need more knowledge to help them understand the problems of *'cystics'* at school, at home and in the working community.

GENERAL PATTERN OF THE ILLNESS

Throughout the body there is a change in the nature of mucous and serous secretions so that the former are abnormally sticky or dry and the latter abnormally concentrated. Much of the pathology results from these characteristics, which allow the secretions to block ducts or ductules. Such obstructions, apparent in a number of organs (Figure 1) are particularly important in the lungs and the pancreas and lead to the cardinal clinical features of CF, which are: **a progressive obstructive suppurative lung disease together with malabsorption due mainly to an insufficiency of pancreatic digestive enzyme secretion.**

In the *pancreas* secretions precipitate within the lumen of the ducts causing blockage and duct dilatation, which on histological section may look like small cysts. Destruction of exocrine pancreatic tissue and replacement with fibrous tissue then occurs. In most cases the alteration of function is already present in the pancreas at birth and therefore clinical evidence of malabsorption is usually, but not always, evident from that time.

The *lungs* are thought to be structurally normal at birth but it

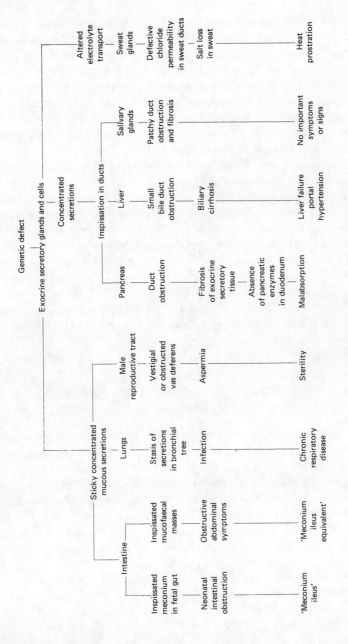

Figure 1. The pathogenesis of cystic fibrosis

appears that the nature of the mucus, secreted by widespread mucous glands in the bronchial tree, allows this mucus to stagnate in the smaller bronchioles. Static secretions become infected. Infection stimulates further mucus secretion and a vicious circle is set up. Infected sticky secretions, difficult to expectorate, become widespread throughout the bronchial tree and produce an obstructive suppurative pulmonary illness. Untreated, this condition is progressive, leading eventually to patchy but widespread bronchiectasis, pulmonary fibrosis and finally to cor pulmonale, cardiac failure and death.

Chronic respiratory disease is the major cause of morbidity and mortality and is the most difficult aspect of the condition to control consistently throughout life. It aggravates considerably the nutritional deficiency caused by malabsorption. It is also possible that pancreatic enzyme insufficiency aggravates the pulmonary condition. **In the untreated patient, therefore, chronic productive cough, dyspnoea, clubbing of the fingers, signs of malnutrition and abnormally greasy offensive stools are the major clinical features.** The severity of these clinical features will vary both intrinsically and with treatment.

The *sweat* is the most obviously abnormal of the serous secretions: its sodium and chloride content is 3–4 times normal. Although serous secretions of other organs, such as the salivary glands, also have a higher than normal electrolyte content, this is not apparent clinically.

HISTORICAL RECOGNITION AND NAMING
OF THE CONDITION

Widespread recognition of CF, despite its importance, has been fairly recent and has developed mainly over the last 50 years. However, some earlier reports are of interest. Landsteiner (1905) described a typical case and included an illustration of the pancreatic histology. Garrod and Hurtley (1912) noted that two members of a sibship of five children, whose parents were first cousins, had had steatorrhoea from early infancy; also that one of these children and another sibling had died with 'bronchopneumonia' and 'bronchitis' at the age of eleven and seven months respectively.

In 1928 Fanconi in Switzerland reported that a group of 'coeliac syndrome' children acquired their symptoms, which included bronchitis, in early infancy. Later, in 1936, he and others recorded the association of 'congenital cystic pancreatic fibrosis' and 'bronchiectasis'.

In 1938 Dorothy Andersen, Pathologist at the Babies' Hospital, New York, gave the first detailed pathological description of the disease. Because of the marked fibrosis and dilated ducts in the pancreas, she termed the disorder 'fibrocystic disease of the pancreas'. She showed the clear association of pancreatic pathology with widespread pulmonary infection and also indicated similar pancreatic changes in newborn infants presenting with intestinal obstruction due to inspissated meconium (meconium ileus). In succeeding years others confirmed these observations and the slightly modified title 'cystic fibrosis of the pancreas' came into use.

In 1945 Sidney Farber in Boston, recognizing the sticky nature of the mucous secretions in the respiratory and alimentary tracts, proposed the name 'mucoviscidosis'.

In 1953 Darling, di Sant'Agnese, Perera and others discovered the high salt content of the sweat and suggested that many or all exocrine gland secretions could be abnormal.

In recent years the name 'cystic fibrosis' or 'CF' has been adopted in most countries. Unfortunately the word 'cystic' gives the misleading suggestion that certain organs of the body are cystic. The name does not give an accurate description of the primary pathology of the disease, which essentially is one of tubular obstruction by thickened secretions, but it must suffice until the elusive basic defect has been discovered.

INCIDENCE

Cystic fibrosis has been described most often in people of European origin, including those who subsequently spread to the Americas, Australia, New Zealand, South Africa etc. However, it is now clear that it is not confined to this racial group although present data show its incidence to be much higher in this group than in others.

Studies in Australia (Danks, Allan and Anderson, 1965), England and Wales (Hall and Simpkiss, 1968; Prosser et al, 1974) and Switzerland (Kaiser, Morer and Hammershlag, 1976) have revealed an incidence of 1:1600 to 1:2300 live births, making CF the most frequent lethal genetic disease among white children. In the United Kingdom, with a population of about 60,000,000 and a birth rate of about 15 per 1,000, some 450 babies with CF are born annually.

There are well documented reports of the condition in children whose racial origins are Negroid, Mongoloid and non-European Caucasoid (Asian-Indian). An incidence of 1:100,000 has been calculated for Monogloid races (Wright, 1969) and 1:17,000 suggested for Negro races (Kulczycki and Schauf, 1974) although a mixture of white and black races, particularly in America, has made it difficult to interpret incidence figures. It is possible that the incidence among Pakistanis and Indians, most of whom are of Caucasoid race, is greater than has been suspected hitherto (Reddy et al, 1969; Goodchild, Insley and Rushton, 1974; WHO, 1985).

INHERITANCE

Inheritance of physical characteristics or diseases is brought about by the transfer of genes from parents to offspring at conception. Genes are located on chromosomes within each cell. They are complex nucleic acids whose structure represents a code or set of instructions which programmes the cells to produce proteins or enzymes. Each gene carries the specific code for a single protein. If neither parent passes on the correct gene for a particular protein to the offspring, that child will be unable to make that protein.

Cystic fibrosis is inherited in an autosomal recessive way, probably as a single locus disease (Romeo, 1984). Both parents 'carry' the abnormal gene, i.e. they are *heterozygotes* who do not have CF themselves. Each child conceived in such a family has a 1:4 chance of inheriting two abnormal CF genes (one from each of his parents) in each of his body cells. If this occurs, he/she will have the disease and will be a *homozygote* for CF. Statistically, in a hypothetical family of four children, two of the remaining three children of such parents will be carriers of the CF gene (i.e. heterozygotes like their parents) and the remaining child will inherit no genes for CF and will be normal both physically and genetically (Figure 2).

Boys and girls have equal chances of being affected. Chromosomal number and appearance are normal. So far, molecular genetic techniques have not identified the defective gene, nor is there any strong evidence for linkage between CF and other disorders or markers (Steinberg et al, 1956; Goodchild et al, 1976; Williamson et al, 1984).

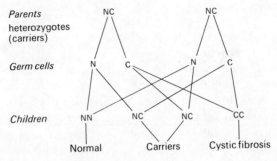

Figure 2. Inheritance pattern

The genetic make-up of the parents is described as NC to show the mixture of normal and CF genes; the make-up of the germ cells (ova and spermatozoa) is described as N or C as a reduction division of the chromosomes takes place in the formation of these germ cells, in order eventually to maintain, in the off-spring, the original chromosome number of the parents; the genetic constitution of the (statistical) four children is shown in the ratio of NN (normal); NC x 2 (carriers); CC (CF)

Gene carrier frequency

From the incidence of the disease in communities of Caucasian origin, the calculated carrier or heterozygote rate is 1:20 to 1:25, making it the highest frequency for an abnormal gene in such a community. As more CF children survive to adult life the genetic risk to their children comes into question. This is not great, partly because CF males are unlikely to reproduce (see Chapter 2). However, even for CF girls, whose fertility is probably only slightly impaired, the chance that they themselves will give birth to CF children is only 1:40 to 1:50, and depends upon whether or not they marry a carrier, or *hetero-zygote*.

The risk of CF in the children of a brother or sister of a CF patient is low and of the order of 1:120 – that is, comparable with the random risk of a major abnormality, of some type, occurring in a child of any 'normal' member of the population.

In a marriage in which only one of the parents is a known carrier (i.e. in second marriages where one of the parents has previously produced a CF child) the chances that this second marriage will result in a CF child is 1:80 to 1:90.

The heterozygote state

Carriers of the gene (heterozygotes) show no symptoms of cystic fibrosis. At present, they cannot be distinguished reliably from non-carriers of the gene although this problem is being actively studied in many laboratories throughout the world.

As CF has been lethal before reproductive age until relatively recently, the existence of a high frequency of carriers in the community has led geneticists to postulate that there is some advantage in being a heterozygote. Some studies suggest an increased birth rate in preceding generations of known heterozygotes (Danks et al, 1965; Knudson, Wayne and Hallet, 1967), but no conclusive evidence for a heterozygote advantage has been presented.

Prenatal screening

Attempts to recognize the CF fetus in early pregnancy, so far, have been more or less confined to pregnancies of parents 'at risk' for CF (i.e. those who have already produced a CF child). A positive prediction would allow an abortion to be considered. Naturally this would not be an acceptable solution to some parents, whether for moral, religious or ethical reasons, but it would be acceptable, or even welcomed by others (Dodge and Ryley, 1982; Kaback et al, 1984).

Considerable effort has been devoted to develop a reliable test. Methods have involved analysis of amniotic fluid obtained from around the developing baby, by needle puncture through the uterus. The most ' encouraging results have come from Edinburgh, UK (Brock, 1983, 1984). Amniotic fluid is procured at 17–18 weeks of pregnancy and the proportion of alkaline phosphatase which is of intestinal origin is measured. This isoenzyme is markedly decreased in amniotic fluid when the fetus has CF.

For babies born into families where a previous child has CF, results have given a high degree of accuracy for prediction of the CF fetus. In other situations (e.g. pregnancies in sibs of known patients, or when only one partner of the marriage is a known carrier – the 'second marriage' situation – or when the mother herself has CF) current tests are not applicable (see page 132).

REFERENCES

Andersen DH. Cystic fibrosis of the pancreas and its relation to celiac disease. A clinical and pathologic study. *Am J Dis Child 1938; 56:* 344–399

Brock DJH. Amniotic fluid alkaline phosphatase isoenzymes in early prenatal diagnosis of cystic fibrosis. *Lancet 1983; ii:* 941–943

Brock DJH. Prenatal screening and heterozygote detection. In Lawson D, ed. *Cystic Fibrosis: Horizons. Proceedings of the 9th International Cystic Fibrosis Congress, Brighton, England.* Chichester: John Wiley. 1984: 1–12

Danks DM, Allan J, Anderson CM. A genetic study of fibrocystic disease of the pancreas. *Ann Hum Genetic 1965; 28:* 323–356

Darling RC, di Sant'Agnese PA, Perera GA et al. Electrolyte abnormalities of the sweat in fibrocystic disease of the pancreas. *Am J Med Sci 1953; 225:* 67–70

di Sant'Agnese PA, Darling RC, Perera GA et al. Abnormal electrolyte composition of sweat in cystic fibrosis of the pancreas. Clinical significance and relationship to the disease. *Pediatrics 1953; 12:* 549–563

Dodge JA, Ryley HC. Screening for cystic fibrosis. *Arch Dis Child 1982; 57:* 774–780

Fanconi G. Der intestinale infantilismus und ahnliche Formen der chronischen Verdaungsstorung. *Jb Kinderkeilk 1928; Suppl 1:* 1–202

Fanconi G, Uehlinger E, Knauer C. Das Coelioksyndrom bei Angeborener zystisher Pankreas fibromatose und Bronchiektasien. *Wein Med Wschr 1936; 86:* 753 –756

Farber S. Some organic digestive disturbance in early life. *J Mich St Med Soc 1945; 44:* 587–594

Garrod AE, Hurtley WH. Congenital family steatorrhoea. *Q J Med 1912; 6:* 242–258

Goodchild MC, Edwards JH, Glenn KP et al. A search for linkage in cystic fibrosis. *J Med Genet 1976; 13:* 417–419

Goodchild MC, Insley J, Rushton DI. Cystic fibrosis in 3 Pakistani children. *Arch Dis Child 1974; 49:* 739–741

Hall BD, Simpkiss MJ. Incidence of fibrocystic disease in Wessex. *J Med Genet 1968; 5:* 262–265

Kaback M, Zippin D, Boyd P et al. Attitudes toward prenatal diagnosis of cystic fibrosis among parents of affected children. In Lawson D, ed. *Cystic Fibrosis: Horizons. Proceedings of the 9th International Cystic Fibrosis Congress, Brighton, England.* Chichester: John Wiley. 1984: 15–28

Kaiser D, Morer HP, Hammershlag P. Experience of 3 years meconium screening in Switzerland. In Hennequet A, ed. *Proceedings of the VII International Congress.* Paris: International CF (Mucoviscidosis) Association. 1976: 148

Knudson AG Jr, Wayne L, Hallet WY. On the selective advantage of cystic fibrosis heterozygotes. *Am J Hum Genet 1967; 19:* 388–392

Kulczycki LL, Schauf V. Cystic fibrosis in blacks in Washington, DC. *Am J Dis Child 1974; 127:* 64–67

Landsteiner K. Darmperschluss durch eingedicktes Meconium Pankreatitis. *Zentralblatt fur allgemeine Pathologie und Pathologische Anatomie 1905; 16:* 903–907

Prosser R, Owen H, Bull F et al. Screening for cystic fibrosis by examination of meconium. *Arch Dis Child 1974; 49:* 597–601

Reddy CRRM, Devi CS, Anees AM et al. Cystic fibrosis of the pancreas in India. *J Pediat 1969; 75:* 522–523

Romeo G. Cystic fibrosis: a single locus disease. In Lawson D, ed. *Cystic Fibrosis: Horizons. Proceedings of the 9th International Cystic Fibrosis Congress, Brighton, England.* Chichester: John Wiley. 1984: 155–164

Steinberg AG, Shwachman H, Allen FH et al. Linkage studies in cystic fibrosis of the pancreas. *Am J Hum Genet 1956; 8:* 162–178

World Health Organization. Cystic fibrosis – a WHO/ICF (M) A meeting. *Bull WHO 1985; 63 (No 1):* 1–10

Williamson R, Gilliam C, Blaxter M et al. Gene cloning – a tool to find the basic defect in cystic fibrosis? In Lawson D, ed. *Cystic Fibrosis: Horizons. Proceedings of the 9th International Cystic Fibrosis Congress, Brighton, England.* Chichester: John Wiley. 1984: 139–153

Wright SW. Racial variation in the incidence of cystic fibrosis. In Lawson D, ed. *Proceedings of the 5th International Cystic Fibrosis Conference.* London: Cystic Fibrosis Research Trust. 1969: 91–102

GENERAL READING

Anderson CM. Cystic fibrosis – the gastrointestinal and nutritional aspects. In Anderson CM, Burke V, Gracey M, eds. *Paediatric Gastroenterology 2nd edition.* Oxford: Blackwell Scientific. In preparation

Doershuk CF, Boat TF. Cystic fibrosis. In Behrman RC, Vaughan VC, eds. *Nelson Textbook of Pediatrics 12th edition.* Philadelphia: W B Saunders. 1983: 1086–1099

Harris CJ, Nadler HL. Incidence, genetics, heterozygote and antenatal detection of cystic fibrosis. In Lloyd-Still JD, ed. *Textbook of Cystic Fibrosis.* Bristol: John Wright. 1983: 1–7

Raeburn JA. Genetics and genetic counselling. In Hodson ME, Norman AP, Batten JC, eds. *Cystic Fibrosis.* London: Baillière Tindall. 1983: 1–12

Talamo RC, Rosenstein BJ, Berninger RW. Cystic fibrosis. In Stanbury JB, Wyngaarden JB, Fredrickson DS, Goldstein JL, Brown MS, eds. *The Metabolic Basis of Inherited Disease 5th edition.* New York: McGraw-Hill. 1983: 1889–1917

Chapter 2

PATHOGENESIS

The pathological changes in cystic fibrosis are notable for their widespread extent and enormous variability. Bodian (1952) published a detailed description of the morbid appearances, which represented the pathology of cystic fibrosis modified only slightly by the treatment available at that time. Earlier descriptions include those of Andersen (1938) and Zuelzer and Newton (1949).

Figure 1 (page 3) illustrates the pathogenesis of cystic fibrosis and relates the final symptomatology to relevant organ pathology. Figure 3 (page 12), a simpler version, shows that clinical features are related chiefly to the alimentary, respiratory and reproductive systems and to the sweating mechanism.

ALIMENTARY SYSTEM

Pathological changes are found in exocrine secretory cells and organs throughout the alimentary tract. The degree of abnormality depends to a large extent on whether the secretions are delivered to the gastrointestinal lumen from cells with narrow necks (such as those of goblet cells), from wide-mouthed ducts (such as those from Brunner's glands in the duodenum) or along narrow ducts and ductules, as found in the pancreas, liver and salivary glands. Narrow, longer ducts are most easily blocked by sticky secretions, resulting in damage to the tissues beyond the blockages. Maximal structural alteration with consequent maximal alteration in function occurs in the pancreas.

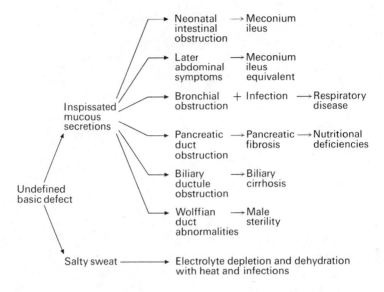

Figure 3. Chief clinical consequences of the undefined basic abnormality in cystic fibrosis

THE PANCREAS

Structural changes

Macroscopic and microscopic changes in the structure of the pancreas are already evident at birth. At this early stage the organ is firmer and more lobulated than normal. Later, the organ becomes much reduced in size, markedly fibrotic and often shows extensive fatty replacement of the parenchyma. Figure 4 illustrates the progression of events — inspissated material in the collecting ducts, damage to acinar tissue, early fibrosis and duct dilatation. Finally there is complete destruction of acinar tissue and replacement by fibrous tissue and fat. Small 'cysts' appear and there is occasional calcification of secretions.

Functional changes

In the majority of patients, these structural changes result in an absence or severe reduction of pancreatic enzymes which digest protein (trypsin

Figure 4. Histological appearance of pancreas in cystic fibrosis illustrating the progression of the changes. (From Hadorn, in Anderson, Burke and Gracey, eds. *Paediatric Gastroenterology*. 1986, with permission)

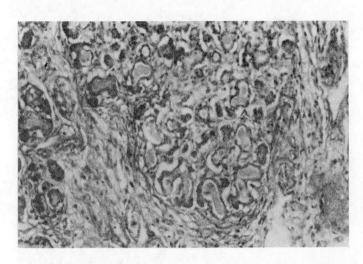

(a) Casts in intercalated ducts (inspissated material stains red with haematoxylin-eosin)

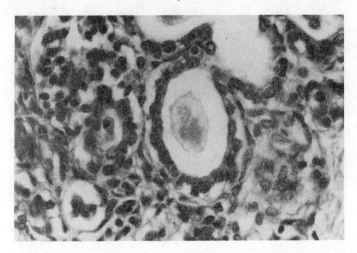

(b) Higher magnification of precipitated material in duct

Figure 4. Histological appearance of pancreas in cystic fibrosis illustrating the progression of the changes. (From Hadorn, in Anderson, Burke and Gracey, eds. *Paediatric Gastroenterology*. 1986)

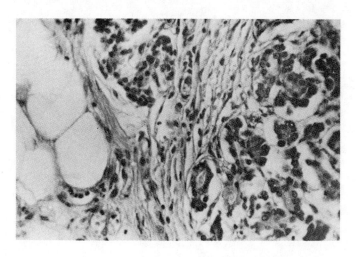

(c) Fibrosis, lipomatous replacement tissue and inspissated secretion in ducts

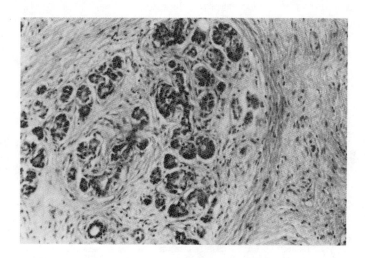

(d) Advanced fibrotic changes

and chymotrypsin), carbohydrate (amylase) and fat (lipase). Consequently proteins are digested inadequately and excess nitrogen is lost in the stools. Starch is incompletely broken down and may appear in the stools as starch grains. The stools are characteristically oily or greasy from undigested fat. Breakdown products of unabsorbed protein produced by bacteria in the large gut contribute towards the offensive smell of stools and flatus.

The insulin-producing cells in *the islets of Langerhans* usually remain normal to light microscopy, although immunofluorescent studies on post-mortem material have suggested that there is a continual process of islet destruction and new cell formation (Kerr, Redmond and Buchanan, 1984). The development of diabetes mellitus in some older patients probably reflects distortion of pancreatic architecture by fibrosis, with impairment of blood supply.

Partial pancreatic insufficiency

Some pancreatic enzyme activity usually remains at birth and evidence from studies of large groups indicates that as many as 10—15 per cent of patients retain some functioning pancreatic tissue throughout life. Investigation of such patients with the use of intravenous pancreozymin shows that enzymes are present, which may even reach normal concentrations. However, all CF patients, whether or not they retain some functioning pancreatic tissue, show a response to intravenous secretin which is grossly impaired, with little or no increase in water and bicarbonate production. This may imply that pancreatic ductular function is abnormal in CF (Hadorn, Johansen and Anderson, 1968).

Pancreatitis

Recurrent attacks of acute pancreatitis have been described in older patients with partial pancreatic insufficiency (Shwachman, Lebenthal and Khaw, 1975). Pancreatic calcification may follow such attacks or on rare occasions it may occur without such an antecedent history.

THE LIVER

Pathological changes occur in the liver and may be present to a minor degree at birth.

Figure 5. Histological appearance of liver in cystic fibrosis

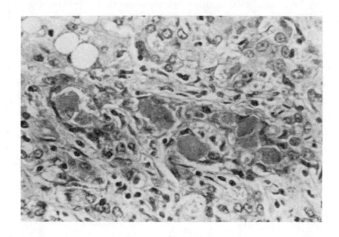

(a) Bile duct plugging in liver of 3-month-old infant – only very small and patchy
    areas of fibrosis seen elsewhere in liver

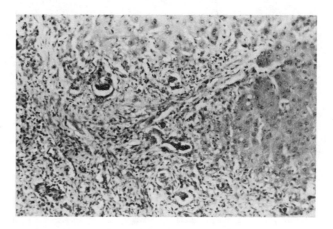

(b) Early periportal fibrosis and multiplication of bile ducts which contain in-
    spissated material

In infants the portal tracts appear prominent and the bile ducts numerous. **Bile plugging occurs in the smaller biliary ductules and there may be scattered areas of fibrosis, pericholangitis and ductule dilatation (Figure 5).** **These changes progress slowly, the rate of progress being very variable and unpredictable.**

Eventually, focal biliary cirrhosis becomes multifocal and, in a few patients, the liver becomes lobulated, hard and shrunken. Fatty infiltration also occurs (Figure 6). Portal hypertension supervenes and haemorrhage from oesophageal varices may be a presenting symptom or a terminal event.

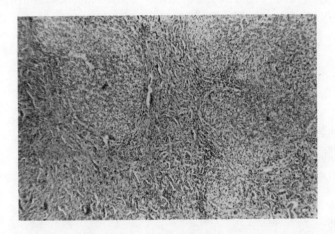

Figure 6. Advanced biliary cirrhosis in 14-year-old boy with cystic fibrosis – note multifocal fibrosis and diffuse fatty infiltration

Biochemical and haematological evidence of liver function does not appear until the cirrhotic changes are well advanced.

Hepatic failure may be the outcome. This is seen only occasionally before late teenage, when it does become more common and affects perhaps 10 per cent of patients.

Unfortunately, as the age of CF patients increases so does the incidence of liver dysfunction and **CF is now an important cause of hepatic cirrhosis and portal hypertension in adolescence and young adults.**

Bile acid metabolism

Bile acids aid the digestion of fats by means of their emulsifying and surface tension lowering properties.

In CF patients with steatorrhoea, there is an excessive loss of bile acids in the stools (Leyland, 1970; Weber et al, 1973; Goodchild et al, 1975). This leads to an interruption of the enterohepatic circulation of bile acids and eventually, a contraction of bile acid pool size (Watkins et al, 1977). With time, a reduction occurs of intraduodenal bile acid concentrations (Harries et al, 1979) with alteration of bile acid type (Goodchild et al, 1975; Harries et al, 1979). These events, together with the pancreatic enzyme insufficiency already present, further impair the digestion and absorption of fat and fat soluble substances; they also make conditions more favourable for the development of gallstones.

If significant *liver disease* is present, the situation may be compounded by an impairment of hepatic bile acid synthesis.

The biliary system

Atresia or obstruction of the cystic duct is frequently associated with a contracted, functionless gall bladder, which contains a small amount of viscid, grey or white mucus (Feigelson, Pecau and Sauvegrain, 1970).

Cholecystitis and cholelithiasis are recorded in children (Kissane and Smith, 1967) and adults (Warwick et al, 1976). The incidence of gallstones increases with age (Warwick et al, 1976) and they are composed almost entirely of cholesterol (Gibbs, 1962; Goodchild, 1980).

OTHER SECRETORY GLANDS

Salivary glands

The degree of abnormality of salivary and buccal glands is related to the mucus content of their secretions. Thus, sublingual and buccal glands ('mucous' glands) show marked retention of secretions, dilatation of acini and some fibrosis; parotid glands ('serous' glands) show minimal change and submandibular ('mixed' glands), an intermediate degree of damage.

Mucous glands and goblet cells of the gastrointestinal tract

Distension of goblet cells is found to a varying degree from oesophagus to rectum (Figure 7a). An irregular layer of 'precipitated' mucus is often present on the surface of the epithelium, particularly in the crypts of the small mucosa (Figure 7b).

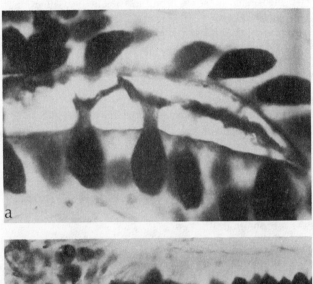

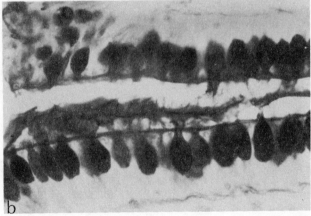

Figure 7 (a) and (b). Small intestinal mucosa in cystic fibrosis illustrating abnormal characteristics of mucous secretions. Note distended goblet cells; mucus extruding from goblet cells; mucus remaining in crypts instead of being dispersed normally. (Acknowledgment is made to D Barry and S Morrissey, for these photographs)

MECONIUM ILEUS

Ten to fifteen per cent of CF babies show symptoms of intestinal obstruction within 24 hours of birth. The small intestinal content, particularly in the ileum, is thick, sticky and dry. This inspissated, dark green meconium, which often contains gas bubbles, fills a varying length of the small intestine, from the jejuno-ileal junction to the ileocaecal valve; on rare occasions it is also found in the ascending colon. The proximal contents are more liquid than the distal contents which may be hard − like rabbit faecal pellets − and adhere to the bowel wall. The bowel is dilated proximal to the blockage and collapsed distal to it, so that the colon appears as a micro-colon which may be filled with white mucus.

Meconium peritonitis occurs occasionally, as a result of antenatal perforation, and flecks of calcium form on the peritoneum and are visible radiologically. Volvulus and atresia complicate about one-third of cases of meconium ileus. The mechanism is likely to be an antenatal twisting of distended bowel, with subsequent alteration of blood supply to the affected loops.

Why is the meconium inspissated?

There are two possible contributory factors: CF meconium has a lower water content and is much more viscous than normal meconium (Griffiths and Watkeys, 1976); there is an increase in albumin and other proteins in CF meconium, owing to deficient pancreatic proteolysis (Harries, 1978; Antonowicz and Shwachman, 1979).

Why do only some CF infants present in this way?

This is not known. At autopsy, shortly after birth, no significant difference has been reported in the degree of pathological change in the pancreas, in CF infants who had had meconium ileus, compared with those who had not (Oppenheimer and Esterley, 1973). In addition, protein contents of meconium have been similar in these two groups (Ryley et al, 1975).

MECONIUM ILEUS EQUIVALENT

In some patients, usually after early childhood, tough, gum-like muco-faeculent masses tend to collect in the caecum or less commonly in the distal ileum. They sometimes become adherent, particularly to the wall of the caecum near the appendix where they may calcify. These masses produce a variety of troublesome symptoms, from bouts of abdominal pain to acute or subacute intestinal obstruction, intussusception, obstructive appendicitis with abscess formation and bowel perforation. The reason for the formation of these masses is obscure. The condition has not been recorded in CF patients without steatorrhoea. It does not appear to be related clearly to the degree of pancreatic insufficiency, although sudden withdrawal of pancreatic supplements, fever and dehydration may precipitate the problem. 'Optimal' treatment of malabsorption with enzymes and perhaps cimetidine, may reduce its incidence (Zentler-Munro, 1983). Meconium ileus equivalent may also follow gastrointestinal infections, when increased amounts of mucus are secreted by the gut.

RESPIRATORY SYSTEM

Both upper and lower respiratory tracts are involved.

Upper respiratory tract

Mucopurulent exudates are found frequently in the nasopharynx, nasal cavities, sinuses and middle ears. Mucosae are congested and acini and ducts of mucous glands are distended. The maxillary antra, in particular, are characteristically opaque on X-ray.

Nasal polyps occur more commonly than in the non-CF patient (Shwachman et al, 1962).

The lungs

Dilation of mucous glands is the earliest feature and possibly the only one present at birth (Andersen, 1962).

In the older, untreated child, stagnation of mucus is followed by infection which stimulates further mucus secretion, producing a vicious circle. Mucopurulent secretions, difficult to cough up, gradually fill the bronchioles and bronchi. Areas of scattered or localized alelectasis develop, alternating with areas of emphysema. Infection gradually destroys the bronchial epithelium and extends into the peribronchial tissues. This leads to peribronchial fibrosis, as well as to weakness of the bronchial walls, with increased dilatation and bronchiectasis which become irregularly scattered throughout the lungs. Erosion of the bronchial walls may result in abscess formation.

In most cases infection spreads very slowly, or sometimes not at all, into the parenchyma of the lungs. Acute bronchopneumonia is rarely seen despite the fact that the *Staphylococcus aureus* is the commonest bacterium isolated from mucopurulent sputum in the patients' early years. The pattern is more that of progressive airways obstruction from retained bronchial secretions and progressive peribronchial fibrosis leading to decreased oxygen/CO_2 exchange. Ultimately, death is usually due to respiratory failure or to cor pulmonale with right heart failure.

With regard to *immunological defence mechanisms,* no specific primary defect has been demonstrated so far (Schiotz, 1982). Inflammatory reaction and antibody response appear to be normal, although it has been suggested, in the case of chronic infection with *Pseudomonas aeruginosa,* that antigen/antibody complexes may enhance pulmonary tissue damage (Hoiby and Schiotz, 1982).

Despite the severity of mucopurulent infection that can arise, this is confined to the lungs and metastatic spread is a rarity. Only a very few cases of systemic amyloidosis in CF have been reported.

The organisms most commonly isolated from purulent secretions are *Staphylococcus aureus* and *Pseudomonas aeruginosa.* In addition, *Escherichia coli* and *Haemophilus influenzae* are common pathogens. During the early years of the recognition of CF in the 1940s and the 1950s, *S. aureus* was the predominant bacterium; now *Ps. aeruginosa* is the one most frequently encountered, particularly among older patients (Mearns, 1980).

At autopsy, the lungs are grossly overinflated and on macroscopic section the bronchioles and bronchi exude thick purulent material. Changes are widespread and never confined to single lobes. Dilatation of bronchi and peribronchial fibrosis is extensive and the walls of pulmonary arteries are thickened.

The lung surfaces may show emphysematous bullae. Occasionally these rupture in life, leading to pneumothorax and pyopneumothorax.

CARDIOVASCULAR SYSTEM

In those dying from the effects of chronic obstructive lung disease, hypoxaemia leads to contraction and hypertrophy of medial muscle fibres in pulmonary arteries and arterioles (pulmonary hypertension). This is followed by right ventricular hypertrophy.

Myocardial fibrosis involving predominantly the *left* ventricle and of uncertain aetiology and relationship to clinical cause, has also been reported.

REPRODUCTIVE SYSTEM

There are several abnormalities in the genital tracts, particularly in the *male.*

Structures derived from the Wolffian duct are poorly differentiated, i.e. the seminal vesicles, vas deferens, epididymis and vasa efferentia. In most patients the vas deferens is atretic or absent, precluding the passage of sperm and this abnormality is present even in the first few months of life. The epididymis is often poorly developed. Testicular histology is usually normal in the prepubertal boy, but testes are sometimes small and immature in the older patient. Spermatogenesis is decreased or absent.

In the female, mucus-producing glands of the cervix uteri may be distended and contain inspissated mucus, this being noticeable in the newborn. Examinations of the endometrium, fallopian tubes and ovaries have been compatible with the patients' ages. Female breast tissue may show lobular agenesis, sparse ducts and ductules and abundant fibrous tissue.

Genesis of these changes

It is not clear whether the anatomical changes are a developmental anomaly of the mesonephric ducts or whether they are analagous to the blockage of ducts which occurs in other parts of the body associated with abnormal secretions. In support of the latter, bulbo-urethral glands have been noted to be distended with mucus and inspissated secretions have been found in the prostate.

URINARY TRACT

Examination of *the kidneys* has shown no very convincing pathological change, although the work of Bodian (1952) and others has suggested an increased incidence of nephrocalcinosis. In the early stages of its development, this calcification seems to be within the lumen of the tubules and to be associated with damage to the epithelial lining. However, at a functional level, the renal handling of certain antibiotics may be altered (see Chapter 5). No consistent defect in electrolyte transport in the tubule has been reported.

SWEAT GLANDS

Despite the high electrolyte content of sweat and the evidence that there is a defect in chloride permeability in the CF sweat duct (Quinton and Bijman, 1983) no structural abnormalities have been described in either the sweat coil or ducts.

OTHER ORGANS

No consistent pathological change as seen by light microscopy has been observed in the central or autonomic nervous systems, lymphoid tissue, exocrine glands, bone marrow, skeletal system, bladder or ureters in younger patients. Minor changes in some of these tissues, probably of a secondary nature, have been seen in older patients — in particular, deficiency of vitamin E has been associated with a peripheral neuropathy, posterior column loss and a myopathy (external ophthalmoplegia) (Tomasi, 1983).

It is clear that the primary structural pathology in this disease is related to abnormalities of exocrine gland secretion.

REFERENCES

Andersen DH. Cystic fibrosis of the pancreas and its relation to celiac disease. A clinical and pathological study. *Am J Dis Child 1938; 56:* 344–399

Andersen DH. Pathology of cystic fibrosis. *Ann NY Acad Sci 1962; 95:* 500–517

Antonowicz I, Shwachman H. Meconium in health and disease. *Adv Pediatr 1979; 26:* 275–310

Bodian M (ed). *Fibrocystic Disease of the Pancreas. A Congenital Disorder of Mucus production — mucosis.* London: Heinemann. 1952

Feigelson J, Pecau Y, Sauvegrain J. Liver function studies and biliary tract investigations in mucoviscidosis. *Acta Paediatr Scand 1970; 59:* 539–544

Gibbs GE. Cholelithiasis in cystic fibrosis. *Cystic Fibrosis Club Extracts, Third Annual Meeting 1962;* 9

Goodchild MC. A study of liver disease in cystic fibrosis, with particular reference to bile acid metabolism. *MD Thesis.* Birmingham. 1980

Goodchild MC, Murphy GM, Howell AM et al. Aspects of bile acid metabolism in cystic fibrosis. *Arch Dis Childh 1975; 50:* 769–778

Griffiths AD, Watkeys JEM. Meconium viscosity in healthy infants and those with meconium ileus. *Biorheology 1976; 13:* 225–230

Hadorn B, Johansen PG, Anderson CM. Pancreozymin-secretin test of exocrine pancreatic function in cystic fibrosis and the significance of the result for the pathogenesis of the disease. *Aust Paediat J 1968; 4:* 8–22

Harries JT. Meconium in health and disease. *Br Med Bull 1978; 34:* 75–78

Harries JT, Muller DPR, McCollum JPK et al. Intestinal bile salts in cystic fibrosis. *Arch Dis Childh 1979; 54:* 19–24

Hoiby N, Schiotz PO. Immune complex mediated tissue damage in the lungs of cystic fibrosis patients with chronic Pseudomonas aeruginosa infection. *Acta Paediatr Scand 1982; Suppl 301:* 63–73

Kerr JI, Redmond AOB, Buchanan KD. Neoformation of islet tissue in cystic fibrosis. In Lawson D, ed. *Cystic Fibrosis: Horizons. Proceedings of the 9th International CF Congress in Brighton, England.* Chichester: John Wiley. 1984: 320

Kissane JM, Smith MG. *Pathology of Infancy and Childhood.* Mosby: St Louis. 1967

Leyland C. Total faecal bile acid excretion in children. *Arch Dis Childh 1970; 45:* 714 (abstr)

Mearns MB. Natural history of pulmonary infection in cystic fibrosis. *Proceedings of the 8th International Cystic Fibrosis Congress, Toronto, Canada.* Toronto: Canadian CF Foundation. 1980: 325–334

Oppenheimer EH, Esterly JR. Cystic fibrosis of the pancreas: morphological findings in infants with and without diagnostic pancreatic lesions. *Arch Pathol 1973; 96:* 149–154

Quinton PM, Bijman J. Higher bioelectric potentials due to decreased chloride and absorption in sweat glands of patients with cystic fibrosis. *N Eng J Med 1983; 308:* 1185–1189

Ryley HC, Neale LM, Brogan TD et al. Screening for cystic fibrosis by analysis of meconium for albumin and protease inhibitors. *Clin Chim Acta 1975; 64:* 117–125

Schiotz PO. Systemic and mucosal immunity and non-specific defense mechanisms in cystic fibrosis patients. *Acta Paediatr Scand 1982; Suppl 301:* 55–62

Shwachman H, Kulczycki LL, Mueller HL et al. Nasal polyposis in patients with cystic fibrosis. *Pediatrics 1962; 30:* 389–401

Shwachman H, Lebenthal E, Khaw KT. Recurrent acute pancreatitis in patients with cystic fibrosis and normal pancreatic enzymes. *Pediatrics 1975; 55:* 86–95

Tomasi LG. Neurological complications in cystic fibrosis. In Lloyd-Still JD, ed. *Cystic Fibrosis.* Boston: John Wright. 1983: 382–408

Warwick WJ, L'Heureux PR, Sharp HL et al. Gallstones in cystic fibrosis. *Proceedings of the 7th International Cystic Fibrosis Congress.* Paris: Imprimerie Jouve. 1976: 484

Watkins JB, Tercyak AM, Szczepanik P et al. Bile salt kinetics in cystic fibrosis: influence of pancreatic enzyme replacement. *Gastroenterology 1977; 73:* 1023–1028

Weber AM, Roy CC, Morin CL et al. Malabsorption of bile acids in children with cystic fibrosis. *N Eng J Med 1973; 289:* 1001–1005

Zentler-Munro PL. Gastrointestinal disease in adults. In Hodson ME, Norman AP, Batten JC, eds. *Cystic Fibrosis.* London: Baillière Tindall. 1983: 144–163

Zuelzer WW, Newton WA. The pathogenesis of fibrocystic disease of the pancreas: a study of 36 cases with special reference to pulmonary lesions. *Pediatrics NY 1949; 4:* 53–69

GENERAL READING

Craig JM, Haddad H, Shwachman H. The pathological changes in the liver in cystic fibrosis of the pancreas. *Am J Dis Child 1957; 93:* 357–369

di Sant'Agnese PA, Talamo RC. Pathogenesis and physiopathology of cystic fibrosis of the pancreas. *N Eng J Med 1967; 277:* 1287–1295, 1343–1352, 1399–1408

Lloyd-Still JD. Meconium. In Lloyd-Still JD, ed. *Textbook of Cystic Fibrosis.* Boston: John Wright. 1983: 153–163

Nezelof C, LeSec A. Multifocal myocardial necrosis and fibrosis in pancreatic diseases of children. *Pediatrics 1979; 63:* 361–368

Oppenheimer EH, Esterly JR. Pathology of cystic fibrosis. Review of the literature and comparison with 146 autopsied cases. *Perspect Pediatr Pathol 1975; II:* 241–278

Reid L. Cardiopulmonary pathology. Perspectives in cystic fibrosis. *Proceedings of 8th International CF Conference, Toronto, Canada.* Toronto: Canadian CF Foundation. 1980: 198–214

Ristow SC, Condemi JJ, Stuard D et al. Systemic amyloidosis in cystic fibrosis. *Am J Dis Child 1977; 131:* 886–888

Talamo RC, Rosenstein BJ, Berninger RW. Cystic fibrosis. In Stanbury JB, Wyngaarden JB, Fredrickson DS et al, eds. *The Metabolic Basis of Inherited Disease 5th Edn.* New York: McGraw-Hill Book Co. 1983: 1889–1917

Chapter 3

CLINICAL AND DIAGNOSTIC FEATURES

INTRODUCTION

Although the majority of patients present in early childhood the **initial diagnosis can be made at any age from birth to adult life.** There is great variability in both the mode of presentation and the severity and progression of the many clinical manifestations, but typical modes of presentation differ according to age.

Table I lists important aspects of the clinical history which are characteristic of the three age groups, while Table II shows the chief features on clinical examination. Table III sets out principal confirmatory investigations. Presentations are described according to age group.

PRESENTATION IN THE NEONATE

Screening procedures may suggest the diagnosis shortly after birth, although a confirmatory sweat test is still necessary. The subject is discussed on page 170.

Ten to fifteen per cent of babies with CF develop symptoms and signs of intestinal obstruction within a few hours of birth. This condition, known as *meconium ileus* is discussed in full on page 108.

PRESENTATION IN EARLY INFANCY

The majority of patients present at this time with a combination of *respiratory symptoms, failure to thrive* and *abnormally offensive,*

TABLE I. Features of clinical history

In the neonatal period	In infancy	Later features
Abdominal distension, bile-stained vomiting and failure to pass meconium, i.e. signs of intestinal obstruction (meconium ileus)	Abnormal stools (usually from birth)	Persistent cough with purulent sputum
	Slow weight gain (usually from birth)	Dyspnoea – at first with exercise only
Occasionally, prolonged neonatal jaundice of obstructive type (present in 50% of cases of meconium ileus)	Large appetite	Recurrent abdominal pain with palpable faecal masses in abdomen, sometimes associated with attacks of subacute intestinal obstruction
	Recurrent or persistent bronchitis	
Testing of meconium for protein content and measurement of immunoreactive trypsin may have been used as screening methods	Noisy, wheezy breathing (secretions in larger airways)	Complications of liver involvement such as haematemesis
	Harsh cough (sometimes paroxysmal)	Progressive thirst, polyuria and weight loss due to diabetes mellitus
	Vomiting with coughing (after paroxysms)	Chronic sinusitis
	Rectal prolapse	Delayed puberty
	'Salty taste' when kissed	Sterility in males
	Rapid finger wrinkling in water	Rarely, symptoms of peptic ulcer
	Family history of deaths in infancy or of living children with similar features	Haemoptysis
	Heat prostration or dehydration in hot weather	

TABLE II. Clinical examination

Early signs	Later signs
Poor growth for age and appetite (use centile chart)	Evidence of malnutrition – progressive if respiratory function deteriorates
Rancid smelling, greasy stools	
Abdominal distension	Increasing evidence of respiratory disease including:
	productive cough
Harsh choking cough	sputum – yellow or green, thick and sticky, often copious
	increasing chest deformity (increase in antero-posterior
Emphysematous shape of chest	diameter and fixity of upper chest)
	lower rib retraction
Increased respiratory rate	variable degrees of cyanosis
	progressive finger clubbing
Persistent lower rib retraction (often slight)	pneumothorax–pyopneumothorax
	pulmonary osteoarthropathy
Evidence of secretions in bronchial tree on auscultation (often minimal)	Nasal polyps and sinusitis
Bronchospasm	Signs of cardiac failure (cor pulmonale)
Early finger clubbing	Liver enlargement (firm, may be irregular)
Dry, pale, mottled skin	Splenic enlargement (signs of portal hypertension)
	Palpable faecal masses in abdomen
Rapid finger wrinkling in water	Delay in development of secondary sexual characteristics

TABLE III. Confirmatory investigations

Test	Initial Findings	Test	Additional Findings
Sweat sodium and chloride – CF levels above 60mmol/L (child) above 70mmol/L (adult)			
Stool microscopy	numerous fat globules	Chemical estimation of fat in faeces	marked steatorrhoea (usually below 50% absorption)
		PABA test	reduction of PABA excretion due to decreased splitting of PABA peptide by chymotrypsin
		Duodenal intubation for pancreatic function	in the majority scanty mucousy juice pH 7 or lower – enzymes and bicarbonate in negligible quantities
			in 10–15% enzyme concentration normal but *bicarbonate and volume very low and juice mucousy*
Chest X-ray	generalized changes — emphysema { horizontal ribs, flattened diaphragm, increased P-A diameter; thickened bronchial markings diffuse patchy consolidation or areas of collapse increasing peribronchial fibrosis		
Cough swab or sputum	Early { *Staphylococcus aureus*, *Haemophilus influenzae*, *Escherichia coli*; Later { *Pseudomonas aeruginosa*, often mucoid strain, *Klebsiella pneumoniae*, *Candida*, *Aspergillus, other fungi*		
Screening tests e.g. meconium albumin, serum immunoreactive trypsin (see page 170)			

bulky, soft and greasy stools. However, *any one of the three* may be the *major feature* or even the only one noted by the parents, and CF should be remembered in the *differential diagnosis of each.*

For example, failure to gain weight may be the only feature noticed by the mother if the patient is her first baby and she is unfamiliar with normal stool characteristics; weight gain may be normal despite pancreatic insufficiency and steatorrhoea, especially if the baby is breast-fed or escapes chest infection until later infancy; in other babies, with only partial pancreatic insufficiency, stools and growth may be normal and chest symptoms may be the only presenting feature. Thus in eliciting a clinical history all such variations should be kept in mind. The view that, 'this baby is too well to have CF' should be discarded.

Very early respiratory signs and symptoms

Many young CF babies present with just a cough which at first is dry and occasional but later harsh and repetitive.

Lung fields may be *clear to examination with the stethoscope* at this early stage but close inspection may reveal any of the following:

slight increase in respiratory rate;
slight increase in antero-posterior diameter and lack of movement of the upper chest;
slight persistent lower rib retraction.

In many babies, in addition to these symptoms, careful questioning will reveal some suggestion of stool abnormality or of poor weight gain, despite a good appetite.

Symptoms and signs of malabsorption in early infancy

(1) Stool abnormalities

In most patients, stools are abnormal from birth; in a few, they become abnormal after several weeks and in a small minority pancreatic enzyme secretion appears to persist throughout life, so that the stools remain clinically normal.

During infancy, stools are characteristically soft, friable, bulky, frequent and highly offensive, having a pungent, cheesy penetrating odour about which the mother may comment, *'You can smell it in the room or toilet even after it has been removed'.* The mother may also say that the stools seem greasy and *nappies are hard to wash clean,* or later, when the stool is passed into a pot, oil — *like melted butter* — oozes from it. If these comments are not made spontaneously by the mother specific enquiry should be made.

Constipation is rare but occurs occasionally in those with only partial pancreatic insufficiency.

(2)   Slow weight gain and large appetite

In many patients, weight increases slowly after birth, progressing below the 25th centile with further delay when chest infection supervenes. In some even gross steatorrhoea makes remarkably little difference to growth in early life and the possibility of the diagnosis may be ignored in the absence of chest infection *if the mother's comments about stool smell and greasy appearance are not taken seriously.* Such infants probably compensate for stool losses by extra calorie intake because of their large appetite, *'his food intake is very good but he does not show much for it'.*

With persistent chest infection there is usually an actual weight loss. The presenting appearance may be that of wasting with obviously thin chest and abdominal walls, and abdominal distension with visible loops of gut.

Despite wasting, physical vigour and normal limb tone usually persist. In fact, CF babies often appear more active than normal babies and seem to require fewer hours of sleep.

Linear growth in the early months is less affected than weight.

(3)   Evidence of protein deficiency

Very occasionally, especially if the infant has been placed on a milk formula low in utilizable protein (such as soya milk preparation) presentation may be with oedema and hypoproteinaemia.

(4)   Evidence of vitamin deficiency

Clinical presentation in this way is rare these days but may occur in babies with pancreatic enzyme insufficiency in whom the diagnosis has been delayed. Only fat soluble vitamins are affected.

Vitamin A deficiency is usually detected by serum measurement but one young infant has been described who presented with a bulging fontanelle (Abernathy, 1976).

Vitamin E Low serum levels are almost universal and the occasional infant may develop haemolytic anaemia or oedema.

Vitamin K CF babies who are particularly prone to a deficiency of this vitamin, causing hypoprothrombinaemia and petechiae, are those who are being breast-fed, who are undergoing surgery or who have concomitant liver disease.

Surprisingly, although *vitamin D* is also fat soluble, clinical evidence of deficiency of this vitamin is rare.

Other suggestive early clinical features

Bronchospasm Some infants may present with bronchospasm and clinical examination may reveal little apart from a few rhonchi. Investigation by chest X-ray, stool examination and sweat test should be considered.

Vomiting This may be an early feature and occurs typically at the end of a bout of repetitive coughing. The *cough* is similar to that of pertussis, para-influenza or other respiratory virus diseases. When there is no epidemic of respiratory viral infection, *such coughing, with or without vomiting, should be considered as due to CF until disproved.*

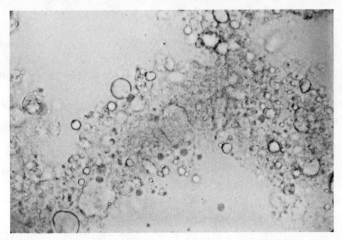

Figure 8. Fat globules in stool of cystic fibrosis patient

Routine investigations

(a) *Stool microscopy* (an easy ward or office procedure). The presence of numerous fat globules (Figure 8) is strongly suggestive of pancreatic enzyme insufficiency and is an indication for relevant chest treatment whilst awaiting a sweat test.

(b) *Chest X-ray.* This may show little except over-inflated lungs with a rather flat diaphragm and, on lateral view, a slightly increased diameter of the upper chest (Figure 9a). Early bronchial thickening, the hallmark of the disease, may be present, together with small scattered areas of infection and/or collapse which are not detectable clinically (Figure 9b).

(c) *Cough swab.* The presence of *Staphylococcus aureus* and/or *Escherichiae coli* is strongly suggestive.

(d) *Sweat test.* This will be confirmatory, but if it is not available quickly, relevant chest treatment should not be delayed: this should do no harm and may possibly prevent the development of irreversible obstructive lung disease.

PRESENTATION IN LATER INFANCY

Cough, vomiting and increased respiratory rate may make sucking difficult and may lead to a decrease in the baby's milk intake. As with the younger infant, failure to thrive with wasting and abdominal distension becomes apparent.

Vomiting may be a feature particularly in the early morning and the presence of purulent sputum in the vomit is very suggestive of the diagnosis of CF.

Other infants present with a history of *intermittent* respiratory symptoms which clear up within a week or two each time. However, after a few months, signs of bronchitic involvement become persistent. Examination of the chest at this stage may reveal widespread moist sounds and X-ray may show widespread patchy areas of consolidation, possibly with segmental or lobar collapse especially in the right upper and middle lobes (Figure 10).

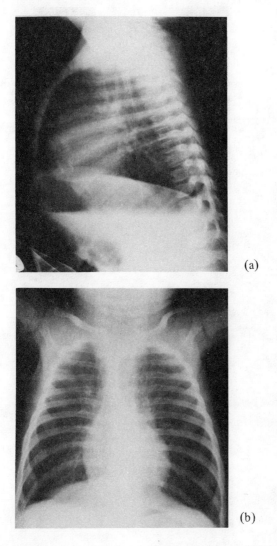

(a)

(b)

Figure 9. Characteristic early changes in chest X-ray appearances of infant with cystic fibrosis: (a) lateral view illustrates emphysematous features – over-distension of lungs (particularly behind the sternum) and low-lying diaphragms; (b) P-A view illustrates typical thickened bronchial wall pattern (most marked medially) and small scattered peribronchial opacities

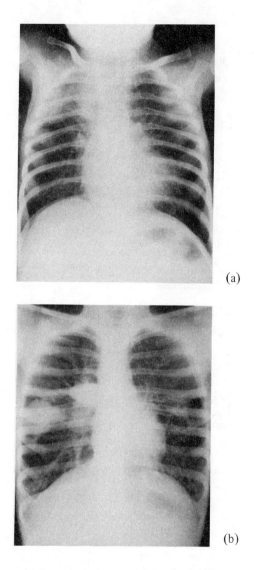

(a)

(b)

Figure 10. Progression of chest disease in cystic fibrosis illustrated by chest X-ray
appearances: (a) P-A view of young infant, showing consolidation and collapse
of right upper lobe and consolidation in the left lower lobe; thickened bronchial wall pattern in other areas; (b) P-A view of older child, showing extensive
bilateral changes and depressed diaphragms. There is consolidation in the
anterior segment of the right upper lobe and in the right middle lobe

Symptoms attributable to salt loss in the sweat in infancy

In hot countries, especially where humidity is high, CF babies (and older patients) may present with 'heat exhaustion' or dehydration with salt depletion.

During the hot New York summer of 1948, 10 cases of heat exhaustion who were treated during a single week were found to have CF (Kessler and Andersen, 1951). The explanation was provided by di Sant'Agnese et al (1953) who recognized the sweat abnormality.

PRESENTATION IN THE TODDLER AGE GROUP

It is less common for the initial diagnosis to be made at this time, but if chest infection is late in appearing, and malnutrition has been slight, the diagnosis may be delayed. Such a child may present with typical features of *malabsorption* or *rectal prolapse*.

Malabsorption syndrome

Abdominal distension and foul-smelling, bulky or frequent stools may be the only obvious features. Coeliac disease (wheat or rye gluten intolerance) may be suspected but the following points should help in differentiating the two conditions.

	Cystic fibrosis	*Untreated coeliac disease*
Stools	Abnormal since birth. Penetrating odour and oily appearance – especially if passed into a pot (melted butter appearance).	Abnormal only after introduction of gluten. Pale but less offensive. No oil seen.
Appetite	Usually very large.	Anorexic or 'difficult' with food.
Personality	Lively, happy.	Quiet, moody, and inactive.
Chest (minor abnormalities)	Increased antero-posterior diameter (slight barrel chest – view sideways), minimal finger clubbing.	No abnormalities.
Stool microscopy	*Numerous fat globules* – some starch grains and meat fibres.	Fatty acid crystals and soapy masses. Very occasional fat globule only.

The features under the heading 'Cystic Fibrosis' indicate sweat test as the next investigation rather than intestinal biopsy for coeliac disease.

Rectal prolapse

This is quite common as a single, presenting symptom in this age group. It is good practice to consider all cases of rectal prolapse in young children as due to CF until proved otherwise. A careful history and examination will often reveal other characteristics of the disease. Although these children may be sent to the surgeon for treatment, medical treatment alone is preferable and usually effective (see page 117).

PRESENTATION DURING SCHOOL AGE

By this time the diagnosis will have been made in the vast majority but a few patients escape detection because chest infections have been absent or minimal. They may present with one or more of the unusual manifestations as set out below.

1. *Meconium ileus equivalent syndrome* — this is a name coined by Jensen (1962) to describe abdominal features including the following:

(a)   recurrent abdominal pain with palpable faecal masses;

(b)   obstructive vomiting and constipation from inspissated faecal masses (Figure 11);

(c)   palpable mass in the right iliac fossa, situated at the ileocolic junction, which may mimic an appendix abscess;

(d)   intussusception — most commonly ileocolic.

2. *Liver enlargement* often presents with a firm, irregular liver and early signs of portal hypertension.

3. *Heat exhaustion* may follow physical exercise in very hot weather.

4. *Diabetes mellitus*

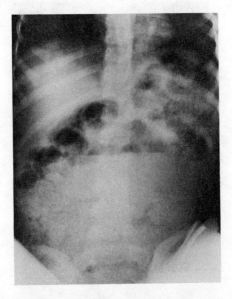

Figure 11. Plain abdominal X-ray (erect film) of 6-year-old child, showing features of the 'meconium ileus equivalent' syndrome — faecal mottling in the colon and fluid levels in the small and large bowel, consistent with a 'blocked' colon

5. *Chronic sinusitis and nasal polyposis*

6. As in the younger groups, *chest infection* can be the presenting feature, previous respiratory involvement being minimal. In these older children chest symptoms and signs may resemble a more classical bronchopneumonic illness. Chest X-ray often shows localized disease such as lobar collapse although generalized changes will be present as well (Figure 12, a and b). With the exceptions of non-CF children who have asthma with infection, or who have inhaled foreign bodies, *lobar collapse is a relatively rare finding in childhood and its presence should raise the suspicion of cystic fibrosis.*

The development of chest disease is very variable, and unpredictable. Even with 'optimal' treatment some cases will deteriorate inexorably, whereas others maintain very good lung function into adult life. Progressive changes are those of increasingly severe obstructive airways disease with emphysema, irregular aeration and a diffusion defect

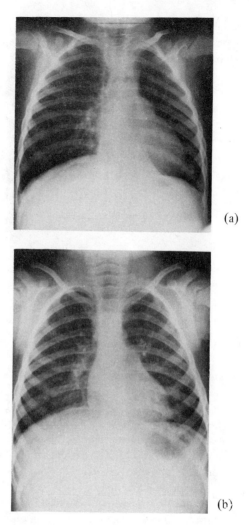

(a)

(b)

Figure 12. Chest X-ray appearances illustrating lobar collapse of the lung in cystic fibrosis: (a) P-A showing complete collapse of left lower lobe; widespread peribronchial opacities in other areas; (b) P-A view 12 months later, showing resolution of left lower lobe collapse. Peribronchial opacities persist and bronchial wall thickening is present in the lingula segment of the left upper lobe

which is discernible by respiratory function tests (see page 173). There is an increase in cough and sputum with the development of barrel-chest, finger clubbing, dyspnoea and cyanosis.

Occasionally, there are episodes of *pneumothorax* or *haemoptysis*. Respiratory insufficiency and right ventricular failure are terminal events. Cardiac failure may be insidious and difficult to diagnose (see page 76).

Chest X-rays, in school age and in the older patient, may show increasing fibrotic change with areas of consolidation and collapse related to fresh upper respiratory tract infections, influenza or measles

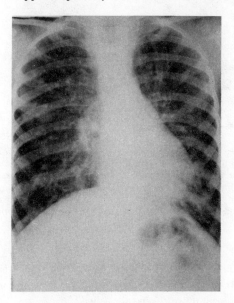

Figure 13. Advanced chest disease in cystic fibrosis. Chest X-ray appearances (P-A view) in 8-year-old child. Note diffuse bilateral changes — multiple linear and nodular opacities

(Figure 13). (Although there is no evidence that CF children are more susceptible to these infections than normal children, the secondary consequences are more important and persistent). On the other hand, remarkably good chest X-rays may be seen, even among the older patients (Figure 14).

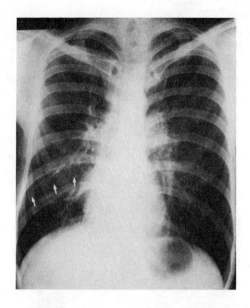

Figure 14. Chest X-ray showing relatively minor changes in a 22-year-old man with cystic fibrosis. There is partial collapse of the right lower lobe (as shown by the depressed transverse fissure — arrows) and some generalized bronchial wall thickening.
This university student has minimal cough and enjoys regular games of squash. His height and weight are on the 90th and 75th centiles respectively

7. Occasionally the diagnosis is made in a *relatively well sib* of a newly diagnosed infant with CF. It is important to perform sweat tests on all sibs of new patients, particularly when minor respiratory symptoms have been present but not taken seriously.

Sputum

The sputum is sticky, thick and *difficult to expectorate*.

If the staphylococcus is the predominant organism the sputum is yellow, but with the advent of pseudomonas, it becomes *green or grey* and more *slimy*, sticking to the sides of a container. Streaks of blood are not uncommon.

PRESENTATION IN ADOLESCENCE OR ADULT LIFE

The *initial diagnosis* is occasionally made in adult life and presentations as late as 46 years (Marks and Anderson, 1960) and 69 years (Evensen, 1981) have been recorded.

The diagnosis may be difficult to confirm as the *sweat test may be more difficult to interpret in these age groups* (Anderson and Freeman, 1960; McKendrick, 1962; Hodson et al, 1983). In addition such patients may now show the full clinical picture and may appear to be less severely affected by the disease being thought, 'too well to have CF'.

Some degree of obstructive pulmonary disease, with digital clubbing, the typical bacteriology, chest signs and chest X-ray appearances, is still the most common mode of presentation, even in adults. However, those who have escaped severe chest disease in youth may be recognized by some of the later, less common characteristics, such as:

(a)   sinusitis and nasal polyposis;

(b)   signs of liver cirrhosis and portal hypertension;

(c)   'meconium ileus equivalent' syndrome;

(d)   recurrent abdominal pain (particularly in those with residual pancreatic function) which may be due to pancreatitis;

(e)   diabetes mellitus;

(f)   growth retardation and delay in sexual development;

(g)   sterility in men due to azoospermia associated in some cases with impalpable vasa deferentia and small testes;

(h)   occasionally reduced fertility in women;

(i)   any of the above features alone or in combination with a suggestive or definite family history.

It is often said that older patients suffer from CF in a milder form and there is evidence that the small proportion who have good pancreatic function with no steatorrhoea have better respiratory function (Gastin et al, 1980).

Investigation in older patients presenting for the first time

Confirmation of diagnosis should not rest on the sweat test alone, as sweat test values increase with age and some values in normal adults may be above 60 or 70mmol/L. However, the diagnosis is strongly suggested when two sweat sodium values are above 70mmol/L and the use of oral fludrocortisone acetate (Florinef) increases discrimination still further (Hodson et al, 1983 see page 163).

The finding of Pseudomonas aeruginosa, particularly of the mucoid variant, is supportive evidence for the diagnosis.

Pancreatic function studies are necessary. Even in the adult, pulmonary and pancreatic components are always there, even if only in minor form.

Before a final diagnosis of CF is accepted, all clinical features and results of investigations should be considered carefully together.

REFERENCES

Abernathy RS. Bulging fontanelle as presenting sign in cystic fibrosis. Vitamin A metabolism and its effect on cerebrospinal fluid pressure. *Am J Dis Child 1976; 130:* 1360–1362

Anderson CM, Freeman M. 'Sweat test' results in normal persons of different ages compared with families with fibrocystic disease of the pancreas. *Arch Dis Childh 1960; 35:* 581–587

di Sant'Agnese PA, Darling RC, Perera GA et al. Sweat electrolyte disturbances associated with childhood pancreatic disease. *Am J Med 1953; 15:* 777–784

Evensen SA. A 69-year-old man with chronic obstructive pulmonary disease, pancreatic insufficiency and elevated sweat electrolytes. *Acta Med Scand 1981; 209:* 141–143

Gaskin K, Gurwitz D, Durey P et al. Improved respiratory prognosis in patients with cystic fibrosis with normal fat absorption. *J Pediatr 1982; 100:* 857–862

Hodson ME, Beldon I, Power R et al. Sweat tests to diagnose cystic fibrosis in adults. *Br Med J 1983; 286:* 1381–1383

Jensen KG. Meconium ileus equivalent in a fifteen-year-old patient wich mucoviscidosis. *Acta Paediat (Uppsala) 1962; 51:* 344–348

Kessler WR, Andersen DH. Heat prostration in fibrocystic disease of the pancreas and other conditions. *Pediatrics 1951; 8:* 648–656

Marks BL, Anderson CM. Fibrocystic disease of the pancreas in a man aged 46. *Lancet 1960; i:* 365–367

McKendrick T. Sweat sodium levels in normal subjects, in fibrocystic patients and their relatives and in chronic bronchitic patients. *Lancet 1962; i:* 183–186

GENERAL READING

Respiratory disease and complications

Hodson CJ, France NE. Pulmonary changes in cystic fibrosis of the pancreas. A radio-pathological study. *Clin Radiol 1962; 13:* 54–61

Holsclaw DS, Grand RJ, Shwachman H. Massive haemoptysis in cystic fibrosis. *J Pediat 1970; 76:* 829–838

Lloyd-Still JD, Khaw KT, Shwachman H. Severe respiratory disease in infants with cystic fibrosis. *Pediatrics 1974; 53:* 678–682

McLoughlin FJ, Matthews WJ, Strieder DJ et al. Pneumothorax: management and outcome. *J Pediatr 1982; 100:* 863–869

Reynolds HY, di Sant'Agnese PA, Zierdt CH. Mucoid Pseudomonas aeruginosa, a sign of cystic fibrosis in young adults with chronic pulmonary disease? *JAMA 1976; 236:* 2190–2192

Stern RC, Borkat G, Hirschfield SS et al. Heart failure in cystic fibrosis. *Am J Dis Child 1980; 134:* 267–272

Gastrointestinal manifestations

Chase HP, Long MA, Lavin MH. Cystic Fibrosis and malnutrition. *J Pediatr 1979; 95:* 337–347

Hanly JG, Fitzgerald MX. Meconium ileus equivalent in older patients with cystic fibrosis. *Br Med J 1983; 286:* 1411–1413

Kulczycki LL, Shwachman H. Studies in cystic fibrosis of the pancreas. 1. Occurrence of rectal prolapse. *N Engl J Med 1958; 259:* 409–412

Nielsen OH, Larsen BF. The incidence of anaemia, hypoproteinaemia, and edema in infants as presenting symptoms of cystic fibrosis: a retrospective survey of the frequency of this symptom complex in 130 patients with cystic fibrosis. *J Pediatr Gastroent Nutr 1982; 1:* 355–359

Roy CC, Weber AM, Morin CL et al. Hepatobiliary disease in cystic fibrosis: a survey of current issues and concepts. *J Pediatr Gastroent Nutr 1982; 1:* 469–478

Shwachman H. Gastrointestinal manifestations of cystic fibrosis. *Pediatr Clin North Am 1975; 22:* 787–805

Stead RJ, Hodson ME, Batten JC. Diabetes mellitus associated with cystic fibrosis in adolescents and adults. *Proceedings of the 12th Annual Meeting European Working Group Cystic Fibrosis, Athens, Greece.* Athens: S Lennis. 1983: 115–118

Valman HB, France NE, Wallis PG. Prolonged neonatal jaundice in cystic fibrosis. *Arch Dis Childh 1971; 46:* 805–809

The condition in adolescents and adults

Anonymous. Cystic fibrosis in adults. Leading article. *Br Med J 1979; 2:* 626

Batten J. Clinical management of the adolescent and adult patient. In *Perspectives in Cystic Fibrosis. Proceedings of the 8th International CF Congress, Toronto, Canada.* Toronto: Canadian CF Foundation. 1980: 183–189

Davis PB. Cystic Fibrosis in adults. In Lloyd-Still JD, ed. *Textbook of Cystic Fibrosis.* Bristol: John Wright. 1983

di Sant'Agnese PA, Davis PB. Cystic fibrosis in adults – 75 cases and a review of 232 cases in the literature. *Am J Med 1979; 66:* 121–132

Hodson ME. Cystic fibrosis in adolescents and adults. Symposium. *Practitioner 1983: 227:* 1723–1731

Mitchell-Heggs P, Mearns MB, Batten JC. Cystic fibrosis in adolescents and adults
    Q J Med 1976; 45: 479–504

Shwachman H, Kowalski M, Khaw K-T. Cystic fibrosis: a new outlook. Seventy
    patients above 25 years of age. *Medicine 1977; 56:* 129–149

Sinnema G, Bonarius JCJ, Stoop JW et al. Adolescents with cystic fibrosis in the
    Netherlands. *Acta Paediatr Scand 1983; 72:* 427–432

Chapter 4

PRINCIPLES OF MANAGEMENT

Management of patients with CF is **complex and varied.**

Treatments must be continued throughout life as none is curative.

Consistent and optimal use of available treatment is important. Inadequate treatment may result in marginal and temporary improvement only, which merely serves to prolong life to some extent, without giving the patient a real sense of well-being.

The clinical care of CF patients involves many factors in addition to the purely medical ones – psychological, social, genetic, educational and occupational. CF becomes an intrinsic part of the life of any family into which an affected child is born, and the patient's doctor to some extent becomes a part of that family. Management is best undertaken by a team of professionals which includes physiotherapists, dietitian, nurses and a social worker as well as medical attendants.

In different parts of the world, many patients with CF are now surviving to go through school life, earn their living, some to marry and bear children – a very different picture from 40 years ago. However, it is still impossible to answer the question, *'what does the future hold for a newly diagnosed infant or child?'*. Intrinsic variations in the disease itself and variations in the degree and type of illness at the time of diagnosis will significantly affect the answer to such a question.

The goal of management and factors affecting its achievement

The objective in management is a child, then adult, who is able to lead a life without undue dependence on others, satisfying to the .

individual and to those near to him. In recent years, an increasing number of CF patients have been able to achieve this.

The following factors play an important part in successful management:

(a)   early diagnosis, ideally at birth, in an asymptomatic state;

(b)   control of chest infection;

(c)   maintenance of adequate nutrition;

(d)   ready availability of knowledgeable medical and ancillary care;

(e)   a family setting where both parents are able to take part consistently with the many aspects of treatment, without undue distress to themselves or to their other children;

(f)   a sympathetic and understanding school environment, where appropriate emphasis is placed on the acquisition of intellectual skills for the CF child;

(g)   the good fortune to avoid the unpredictable, and largely unpreventable, complication of liver cirrhosis;

(h)   optimal control of other complications such as diabetes mellitus and meconium ileus equivalent;

(i)   the ability of the patient to come to terms with his condition, particularly during the difficult period of adolescence, when so many patients discontinue various aspects of treatment, notably physiotherapy;

(j)   the acceptance by the community at large of the limitations which the condition necessarily imposes.

While longevity depends to a large extent on the maintenance of adequate pulmonary function and nutrition, there are several other facets. General principles of management are discussed in the next few paragraphs and treatments relating to individual systems are set out in succeeding chapters (Chapters 5–8).

FEATURES OF MANAGEMENT COMMON TO ALL PATIENTS

Achievement of a normal life style whenever possible

Physical activity, both at home and at school, should be restricted only by the patient's tolerance.

A normal education at a normal school should be the aim for the majority. Intellect in these children is unimpaired and they often have an unusually high aptitude for sustained mental and physical effort.

Parental and patient education

The management of CF and its implications for the life of the child and his family should be explained, and reinforced by further discussion. The young patient should be encouraged to accept his disease, from his early years. Eventually, most patients come to understand their condition very fully and take the initiative correctly in the treatment of their problems.

Immunizations

Immunizations against diphtheria, tetanus, pertussis and poliomyelitis should be performed at appropriate ages with the usual exceptions and precautions. Booster doses also should be given as for normal children. Sibs too, should be protected whenever possible, so that they do not convey the infections actively to the CF child.

Live vaccination against measles is strongly advised as its pulmonary complications may be serious. The vaccine should be given when the child is as well as possible, but is not contraindicated by mild, chronic chest disease.

In the event that the unvaccinated CF child is exposed inadvertently to measles, an injection of *normal immunoglobulin* may be given, *preferably within 24 hours in order to prevent an attack, or within seven days to modify one.* If measles does not develop, the injection should continue to act as a deterrent for three months, when the active vaccine should be given. This active vaccine would not be detrimental to the child if measles had developed in modified form, but was unrecognised clinically; indeed, in these circumstances, the vaccine should be given.

Measles vaccine is usually given at about the age of one year, but if it has been omitted at this age, it may still be valuable to give it up to the age of five years.

Ideally, *influenza vaccine* should only be recommended if the particular virus responsible for an epidemic could be identified and an appropriate vaccine made available. However it is common practice to give influenza vaccine on an annual basis to older children (i.e. over the age of four years) attending cystic fibrosis clinics. This probably offers protection against about 60 per cent of outbreaks of influenza which may be encountered. It is perhaps important that the 'very well' patient should be protected because an attack of influenza may precipitate the first severe chest illness. Sometimes it can also cause exacerbations in patients with established respiratory disease.

Dietary salt

In hot and humid countries in particular, this should be given in order to offset the increased salt loss in sweat which is approximately four times normal. In normally cool countries, the mother should be advised on the need for added salt when unusual heat waves occur. Details of dosage etc., are given in Chapter 7, page 124.

Fluids and electrolytes during febrile illnesses

Any CF patient requiring intravenous fluids, for whatever reason, is likely to have an unusually high requirement for sodium and potassium. Unless the attendant is aware of this, quite depleted levels may occur. Infants, in particular, may develop quite severe metabolic alkalosis, with depletion of sodium, potassium and chloride. The provision of adequate electrolytes will usually rectify the situation.

Contact with infections

Close contact with individuals *with acute upper respiratory infections* should be avoided if possible but not carried to the extreme of altering the patient's usual life pattern.

There is no evidence that cystic fibrosis patients are more susceptible to the common cold, to other viral respiratory infections or to other infectious diseases than their sibs; often they seem to be less so.

The condition is not infectious

Despite the presence of *Staphylococcus aureus, Pseudomonas aeruginosa* and other organisms in the respiratory secretions, cross infection to friends and to normal sibs rarely occurs.

It should be made clear to the school that the child's cough is not infectious.

Hospital admissions

Unless admission is required for expert physiotherapy, or simply to give the parents a rest, hospital admissions should be kept to a minimum. Straightforward diagnostic procedures can be carried out from the outpatient department or on a day basis. An ill patient of course will need admission but once treatment is established and improvement occurring, this can be continued at home if parents are adequately instructed (e.g. the administration of antibiotics for the treatment of pseudomonas chest infection (see page 65).

If the patient is the first CF child in the family and the mother needs support and reassurance, it may be necessary to initiate the treatment regime in hospital, even in a relatively well child. However, the stay in hospital should not be prolonged unnecessarily. Home care may avoid the possibility of exposure to other infections and other antibiotic-resistant organisms.

Regular review

Review by a paediatrician experienced in the care of CF children is essential. We review children under the age of 12 months at monthly intervals, and older 'average' patients approximately each three months, the time interval varying according to the clinical need.

ASSESSMENT OF THE VALUE OF INDIVIDUAL
ASPECTS OF TREATMENT

It is clearly important to work out systems by which individual aspects of treatment can be assessed, particularly in the long term. This is not easy because of a number of problems: ethical considerations; intrinsic variations in the severity of the disease between individuals; the natural progression of the disease; the complex nature of treatments, with possible changes in personnel; environmental variations, of infection for example, which are likely to occur during the course of the study; difficulties in assessing the results of any new treatment in the absence of the criterion of cure.

Nevertheless, well-designed trials of new medications or other approaches to treatment are constantly in progress. For example, in the case of a drug trial, the optimal format is a double-blind, placebo controlled cross-over trial in which neither the patients nor the assessors know whether active drug or placebo is being given. However, before embarking on comparisons of treatment it is essential to obtain the advice of a medical statistician to ensure the best trial design.

GENERAL READING

Anderson CM. Long-term study of patients with cystic fibrosis. *Bibl Paediat 1967; 86:* 344–349

Beckerman RC, Taussig L. Hypoelectrolytemia and metabolic alkalosis in infants with cystic fibrosis. *Pediatrics 1979; 63:* 580–583

Dinwiddie R; Redmond AOB; Hodson ME; Littlewood JM. Cystic fibrosis: Special report. *The Practitioner 1980; 224:* 291–294; 295–299; 301–303; 305–307

di Sant'Agnese PA, Davis PB. Cystic fibrosis in adults. 75 cases and a review of 232 cases in the literature. *Am J Med 1979; 66:* 121–132

Williams AJ, McKiernan J, Harris F. Heat prostration in children with cystic fibrosis. *Br Med J 1976; 2:* 297 (letter)

Wilmott RW, Tyson SL, Dinwiddie R et al. Survival rates in cystic fibrosis. *Arch Dis Childh 1983; 58:* 835–836

Chapter 5

MANAGEMENT OF RESPIRATORY DISEASE

For most patients, respiratory disease is the most serious manifestation of cystic fibrosis and the rate of its progression determines the well-being and life span of the individual.

Control of infection and removal of thickened bronchial secretions are the primary goals of treatment and are attempted by:

1. **the administration of antibiotics;**

2. **chest physiotherapy with coughing, breathing exercises, postural drainage and exercise.**

Other forms of treatment include intermittent inhalation of moisture, antibiotics, mucolytic agents or bronchodilators.

The administration of antibiotics is of limited value without effort to remove bronchial secretions by physiotherapy and the two should go hand in hand.

ADMINISTRATION OF ANTIBIOTICS

General principles

Although it is difficult to separate the beneficial effect of the various aspects of treatment, longer survival and improved quality of life have been associated with the advent of antibiotics, especially the penicillinase-resistant and cephalosporinase-resistant (i.e. beta-lactamase-resistant) varieties. However, there are still considerable differences of opinion as to *when and for how long antibiotics should be given.*

The following are common practices:

1. continuous antibiotic therapy, using a narrow spectrum, anti-staphylococcal agent from the time of diagnosis throughout life; additional antibiotics used intermittently as required;

2. *continuous therapy, with an antistaphylococcal agent for the early years only; again, additional antibiotics used intermittently as required;*

3. intermittent therapy at all ages, using various antibiotics, singly or in combination, guided by what appears to be the clinical need.

Sometimes, deterioration of health on intermittent therapy necessitates change to a continuous regime. In all cases, usage of antibiotics should be monitored against changing organisms and changing sensitivity.

Detailed controlled studies to show which regime is most effective are not available. Short-term studies are of little value and long-term studies are subject to enormous variables (see Chapter 4).

Some arguments in favour of using a continuous antibiotic (in particular, an antistaphylococcal agent) from the time of diagnosis, which should be as early in life as possible, are discussed below.

1. CF lungs are considered to be structurally normal at birth (Andersen, 1960) and are likely to be normal to lung function tests also (Beardsmore, Godfrey and Katznelson, 1983).

2. Serial lung function tests indicate the progressive nature of cystic fibrosis even in the young child (Phelan et al, 1969; Godfrey, Mearns and Howlett, 1978) and mortality may be significant, even in the first three months of life (Lloyd-Still, Khaw and Shwachman, 1974).

3. Improved survival curves in recent years indicate that some aspect(s) of treatment (not necessarily antibiotics alone) must have played a part in this improvement. Greatest reductions in mortality have been during the first year of life (Anderson, 1967; Nielsen and Schiotz, 1982; Wilmott et al, 1983).

4. The staphylococcus remains perhaps the most important pathogen in the child's early years (Burns and May, 1968; Mearns, Hunt and Rushworth, 1972).

5. Continuous treatment of CF patients with the antistaphylococcal agent, cloxacillin, showed that no antistaphylococcal precipitins were detected in the CF patients, in comparison with rising levels found among normal, untreated children with increasing age (McCrae and Raeburn, 1974; Lawson and Porter, 1976) — suggesting that staphylococcal growth in the CF patients had been controlled by treatment.

Other arguments are against the continuous use of an antibiotic, including an antistaphylococcal agent.

A number of observations have suggested that prolonged continuous therapy may predispose towards the colonization of CF lungs with *Pseudomonas aeruginosa*, which is impossible to eradicate and associated with considerable lung damage. The evidence is as follows.

1. Since the 1950s, when many physicians began to give antistaphylococcal agents, a decline has been noted in the rate of isolation of the staphylococcus from the sputum of CF patients, with an increase in the isolation of pseudomonas (Mearns, 1980).

2. While *Staphylococcus aureus* and *Haemophilus influenzae* remain the most common pathogens in the young child, *Pseudomonas aeruginosa* becomes more frequent with increasing age (Mearns, Hunt and Rushworth, 1972; May, Herrick and Thompson, 1972).

3. The studies of Kulczycki, Murphy and Bellanti (1978) and Kulczycki et al (1984) suggest that prolonged use of antibiotics may encourage the development of pseudomonas colonization and the appearance of mucoid strains.

However, these studies do not rule out the existence of a group of CF patients who are more susceptible to colonization with pseudomonas and there are numerous incidences of young children with pseudomonas cultured during their initial respiratory infection.

These observations, therefore, present the clinician with a dilemma. Clearly, some aspects of antibiotic treatment during the last 40 years have been beneficial, but not all.

The young child poses a special problem because of his narrow airways, limited ability to co-operate with physiotherapy and inhalations and possibly, because of his increased liability to upper respiratory tract infections. Moreover, during the first two years or so the lungs are still developing in complexity and not merely growing in size.

Thus it would seem particularly important to pay special attention to the young CF child so that he reaches school in a good state of health, not too different from his peers, and able to co-operate with the treatment regime.

For *older school children* the problem should be simpler. By this time the patients and parents are more familiar with the condition, children are more co-operative, physiotherapy is more efficient, bronchial passages are larger and children take more of the types of physical exercise which are helpful in clearing the lungs of secretions. Upper respiratory tract infections are less frequent after early school years.

Should therapy be intermittent at all ages, guided by what appears to be the clinical need?

On account of the foregoing paragraphs we suggest that while this may be a sensible compromise for the school age and older patient, it may not be the best approach for the pre-school child.

In common with many paediatricians holding CF clinics in Great Britain, we use the following regime:

continuous antibiotic (antistaphylococcal) treatment, using a single agent for the pre-school and possibly the early school years; additional antibiotics as required; intermittent therapy, only, as required for the subsequent years and adult life.

However we believe that of even greater importance than the actual regime employed is the need for frequent outpatient surveillance of the young child, in order to start treatment, if this seems important, early in the development of a respiratory infection.

FACTORS GOVERNING THE CHOICE OF ANTIBIOTICS

Identification of pathogens in respiratory secretions

Samples obtained from a cough swab do not necessarily reflect the bacteriology of the lungs, but may be the only ones obtainable. Cultures are made from sputum or a cough swab and a variety of media are chosen with the expected organisms in mind. Sensitivities of possible pathogens are then determined to a broad range of antibiotics. Cultures should be repeated at each clinic visit.

Taking a cough swab

This should be done by someone practised in the art who realizes that information is being sought on the bacterial content of lung secretions and not just of mouth flora.

The swab should be taken during coughing so that a blob of mucus or mucopurulent material can be collected.

If obtainable, *sputum* should be used for culture rather than a throat swab.

Bacteriology of bronchial secretions

Staphylococcus aureus is the organism most commonly present in early pulmonary infection and is thought to be the primary invader, others following after it has become established. It may also be found in the culture of a throat swab from the infant without a cough. Serum precipitins to the staphylococcus appear early in the disease; precipitins to the other organisms follow later. The predilection of *Staphylococcus aureus* for the bronchial secretions of CF patients has never been explained satisfactorily.

Haemophilus influenzae may be an important early pathogen, which may persist. Like *Staphylococcus aureus* it may be overlooked when culture plates are overgrown with *Pseudomonas aeruginosa* unless selective media are used.

Escherichia coli, *Klebsiella pneumoniae* and *Proteus species* are found occasionally.

Pseudomonas aeruginosa is a later invader and more common in those with progressive chest involvement. Two varieties are found: a 'mucoid' type which has an extracellular coating of mucopolysaccharide and a 'non-mucoid' type which does not have this coating (see Figure 15). The 'non-mucoid' form is commonly found when chest infection is still relatively minor and it converts quickly, within the environment of the CF lung to the 'mucoid' form. Both types of pseudomonas are associated with a progression of chest infection and with thickened, viscous, green or grey sputum.

The presence of the 'mucoid' form is almost unique to cystic fibrosis and it may even suggest the diagnosis (Reynolds, di Sant'Agnese and Zierdt, 1976). The reason for this is unknown. In the laboratory, the 'mucoid' form will revert to the 'non-mucoid' if transferred serially

Figure 15

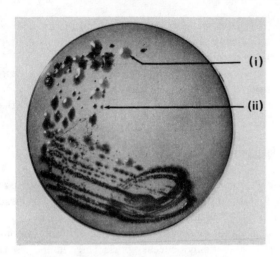

(a) Culture plate to show colonies of *Pseudomonas aeruginosa,* both 'mucoid' (arrow, i) and 'non-mucoid' (arrow, ii)

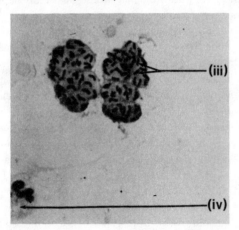

(b) Gram-stained *Pseudomonas aeruginosa* bacteria (arrow, iii) with surrounding mucopolysaccharide coating. A white blood cell with nucleus (arrow, iv) is included to indicate comparative size. (Acknowledgment is made to Mr A Paull, Department of Medical Microbiology, University Hospital of Wales, Cardiff, for these photographs)

(Zierdt and Schmidt, 1964). Other bacteria within the CF lung, for example *E. coli,* may also acquire a 'mucoid' coating, of a different biochemical and antigenic type (Macone et al, 1981).

Mechanisms by which the pseudomonas produces pulmonary damage are not fully understood, but include the effects of exotoxins and proteases produced by the bacterium (Bergan, 1981) and immunological responses (Marks, 1981; Hoiby and Schiotz, 1982).

Once the CF lung is colonized with the pseudomonas it is impossible to eradicate. However, this does not allow a prediction to be given for the outlook of that individual; while in some it appears to herald a clinical deterioration, in others the pseudomonas may be present for 20 years or more before a serious debilitating lung infection occurs.

Apart from *Pseudomonas aeruginosa* other pseudomonads (e.g. *Pseudomonas cepacia)* have been seen in recent years, particularly in CF clinics in Canada and North America (Isles et al, 1984). This variety seems to be rather resistant to treatment.

On very rare occasions, Legionella pneumophilia, Mycobacterium tuberculosis, and other mycobacteria and anaerobic species, may act as pathogens. In the compromised host, in particular, *Mycoplasma pneumoniae* and chlamydia may be important. Fungal infection may also occur (see page 70).

USE OF PARTICULAR ANTIBIOTICS

Antistaphylococcal antibiotics

As recommended earlier in this chapter, these should be given in therapeutic dosage from the time of diagnosis and during the early pre-school years, even in the absence of symptoms and signs of chest disease and in the absence of *Staphylococcus aureus* from the cough swab. It is known from autopsy material that peripheral bronchial secretions will almost certainly contain this organism.

Flucloxacillin is one of the effective antibiotics for long-term use against *Staphylococcus aureus* and side effects are few (Table IV). Resistant strains of *Staphylococcus aureus* rarely occur. The occasional child will refuse it because of its bitter tase. In these or in children allergic to penicillin, **erythromycin is a useful alternative, but resistant strains are more likely to emerge.**

TABLE IV. Oral and systemic antibiotic therapy in cystic fibrosis — suggested drugs (in alphabetical order), dosages and comments

(A) ORAL PREPARATIONS

Drug	Amount per dose (q.d.s. unless stated otherwise)			Comments
	During 1st year (10–25% adult dose)	1–7 years (25–50% adult dose)	7 years + (50–100% adult dose)	
Amoxycillin	125mg t.d.s.	250mg t.d.s.	250–500mg t.d.s.	Useful against some Gram-negative organisms, especially *H. influenzae*. Rashes and loose stools may occur. Amoxycillin better absorbed.
Ampicillin	125mg	250mg	250–500mg	
Chloramphenicol	12mg/kg (avoid in neonates)	125mg	250mg	'Broad spectrum' antibiotic occasionally used. 'Hospital staphylococcus' may be sensitive. Aplastic anaemia and optic neuritis are rare complications (see page 64).

(continued on next page)

(A) ORAL PREPARATIONS

Drug	Amount per dose (q.d.s. unless stated otherwise)			Comments
	During 1st year (10–25% adult dose)	1–7 years (25–50% adult dose)	7 years + (50–100% adult dose)	
Cotrimoxazole	4mg/kg b.d.	40–80mg b.d.	80–160mg b.d.	Dose expressed as trimethoprim. Useful broad-spectrum alternative to amoxycillin. Side effects including rashes, erythema nodosum less likely with trimethoprim (see below)
Erythromycin	125mg	250mg	250–500mg	Alternative anti-staphylococcal agent, also effective against *H.influenzae*. E. stearate should be used rather than E.estolate, as latter can produce cholestasis.
Flucloxacillin	125mg	250mg	250–500mg	Prophylactic and therapeutic anti-staphylococcal agent. Often used in combination with amoxycillin or erythromycin. Bitter taste.

(continued on next page)

(A) ORAL PREPARATIONS

Drug	Amount per dose (q.d.s. unless stated otherwise)			Comments
	During 1st year (10–25% adult dose)	1–7 years (25–50% adult dose)	7 years + (50–100% adult dose)	
Fusidic acid	12.5mg/kg as the acid 15mg/kg as the sodium salt	15mg/kg as sodium salt	250–500mg as sodium salt	Antistaphylococcal. May be used in conjunction with flucloxacillin. Suspension contains 250mg fusidic acid in 5ml. One capsule is approximately equivalent to 7.5ml suspension. Liver function should be monitored with prolonged usage.
Sodium fusidate (see fusidic acid)				
Tetracyclines	–	–	250–500mg	Useful broad-spectrum antibiotic, especially for *H.influenzae* and mycoplasmas. Avoid in children under 12 years.
Trimethoprim	4mg/kg b.d.	50–100mg b.d.	100–200mg b.d.	Broad-spectrum. See co-trimoxazole.

(continued on next page)

(B) SYSTEMIC PREPARATIONS

Drug	Amount per dose	Comments
Aminoglycosides	*For normal renal function in* *a) children:*	Effective against *Ps. aeruginosa* and other Gram-negative organisms. Usually used in combination with appropriate penicillin or third generation cephalosporin (but administered serum separately). Monitor serum drug levels and serum creatinine (see page 67).
Gentamicin	2.5 – 3 mg/kg 8 hourly	
Netilmicin	4 mg/kg 12 hourly (can be 8 hourly)	
Tobramycin	2.5 – 3 mg/kg 8 hourly	
	b) in adults:	
Gentamicin	80 – 120 mg 8 hourly ⎫ adjust	
Netilmicin	150 mg 12 hourly ⎬ according	
Tobramycin	80 – 120 mg 8 hourly ⎭ to drug levels	
Penicillins		Antipseudomonas and broad-spectrum. Used in combination with an aminoglycoside. Must be I.V., bolus by slow injection or short infusion. Dilute as recommended by manufacturers. Drip site should be inspected daily for 'allergic' reactions and venous thromboses.
Azlocillin	Child: 75 – 100 mg/kg 8 hourly	
	Adult: 2 – 5 g 8 hourly	
Carbenicillin	Child: 100 mg/kg 6 hourly	
	Adult: 5 g 6 hourly	
Ticarcillin	Child: 76 mg/kg 6 hourly	
	Adult: 4 g 6 hourly	
Third generation *cephalosporins*		Very effective against *Ps. aeruginosa* and other Gram-negative organisms. Often used in combination with an aminoglycoside. Preferably I.V., bolus or infusion; should be well diluted (as recommended by manufacturers). Inspect drip site for local reactions.
Ceftazidime	Child: 30 – 50 mg/kg 8 hourly	
	Adult: 1.5 – 2 g 8 hourly	

Other antibiotics may be used, probably in conjunction with flucloxacillin, for the treatment of staphylococcal chest infection. These include, **fusidic acid** (caution in the presence of recognized liver disease) and **chloramphenicol** (see below).

Cephalexin is probably not ideal as this may engender resistance in later life to cephalosporin derivatives which are active against *Pseudomonas aeruginosa.*

Cotrimoxazole (Septrin, Bactrim). This is a useful agent, often given in combination with flucloxacillin and is effective against a range of organisms, including not only the staphylococcus but *Haemophilus, Proteus* and *Escherichia* species.

Tetracyclines are broad spectrum drugs, active against the majority of Gram-positive and Gram-negative bacteria, exept for most strains of proteus and of course, *Pseudomonas aeruginosa.* They are also useful against mycoplasmas.

As for all children, they should not be given under the age of 12 years or to pregnant patients, on account of their ability to discolour developing teeth.

Treatment of *Haemophilus influenzae* and other Gram-negative organisms

The decision to treat these is often difficult. *Haemophilus influenzae* is more likely to be an active pathogen than many other Gram-negative bacteria. Isolation from sputum is probably more significant than from a cough swab and if the child remains unwell, these organisms should be treated on the basis of sensitivity tests.

Amoxycillin (a derivative of ampicillin, showing improved absorption and some reduction of gastrointestinal side effects), **erythromycin** and **cotrimoxazole** are the mainstays. All may be given in combination with flucloxacillin.

Dosages of amoxycillin commonly given, over two to three weeks, are on Table IV, but one report (Knight, 1983) advocates much larger doses (3g b.d. for adults) for several weeks or months.

Tetracyclines are effective also.

Chloramphenicol is infrequently recommended because of the risks — the extremely rare development of aplastic anaemia in sensitive subjects and of optic neuritis if the dose exceeds 50mg/kg/day for longer than two to three months (Huang et al, 1966) — but occasions can arise in the treatment of CF when potential benefits outweigh the risks.

Chloramphenicol is active against a wide range of bacteria including most of the gram-negative bacilli of clinical significance.

Side effects from all these antibacterial agents are few. Some patients, particularly infants, develop loose stools and perianal soreness, usually attributable to flucloxacillin or amoxycillin. This may respond to reduced dosage or to change of antibiotic.

Oral and perineal thrush is sometimes responsible for the soreness and this usually clears up with topical nystatin, miconazole or amphotericin, together with reduction of the combined antibiotic dosage or its frequency.

Treatment of *Pseudomonas aeruginosa*

This organism, once it is established in CF lungs, is impossible to eradicate, even for brief periods. However, when it is associated with symptoms, treatment can produce very worthwhile clinical improvements.

The decision to treat it will depend on a number of factors — whether the patient is 'well' or 'ill' (weight change and appetite are important markers); whether sputum has increased in volume, darkened in colour and become more viscous; whether chest signs and chest X-ray changes have become more substantial. An 'incidental' finding of the bacterium, on a routine culture, does not necessarily indicate treatment.

Most CF patients, especially the older ones, live 'in balance' with their pseudomonas, requiring treatment at intervals — this may vary from once to four or more times per year and the pattern tends to be characteristic of that individual.

Once the bacterium is established, some authorities encourage treatment on a regular, three-monthly basis, reporting better survival (Szaff, Hoiby and Flensborg, 1983) while others prefer to treat according to symptoms and individual requirements.

Regarding the manner of treatment, this remains largely by intravenous injection and infusion which may be either in hospital, or, after insertion of the cannula and suitable instruction, at home (Winter et al, 1984).

There are many anti-pseudomonal agents and any one patient is unlikely to have organisms resistant to all, or to most of them.

Another approach to treatment is *by inhalation* either in conjunction with intravenous treatment, or by itself. Although somewhat cumbersome and time-consuming inhalations can be effective, improving health and reducing hospital admissions (see page 68).

Oral anti-pseudomonal agents are being developed and are undergoing trials. At the moment, these are quinolone derivatives and are active against a wide range of organisms, including *Pseudomonas aeruginosa* (Editorial, 1984).

The effectiveness of a *polyvalent pseudomonas vaccine* has been studied, but so far this did not prevent colonization with *Pseudomonas aeruginosa* and did not modify the progress of the disease (Langford and Hiller, 1983).

Drugs available for the treatment of Pseudomonas aeruginosa

Those currently available fall into four main groups:

aminoglycosides e.g. gentamicin, tobramycin, netilmicin, amikacin;
ureidopenicillins e.g. azlocillin, mezlocillin, piperacillin;
carboxypenicillins e.g. ticarcillin, carbenicillin;
third generation cephalosporins e.g. ceftazidime, cefsulodin.

The last three groups, particularly the third generation cephalosporins are relatively beta-lactamase resistant although organisms with beta-lactamases active against these antibiotics are now encountered.

The best remissions are probably achieved with a *combination of antibiotics* which act synergistically and perhaps prevent the emergence of resistant strains.

Effective combinations are an aminoglycoside together with either a ureidopenicillin or one of the third generation cephalosporins.

Gentamicin and **tobramycin** are equally effective at a practical level (Hodson, Wingfield and Batten, 1983) although it has been reported that tobramycin is less nephrotoxic but equally ototoxic (Smith et al, 1980). **Netilmicin** is probably less ototoxic than tobramycin and can be given twice daily (Lerner et at, 1983).

Azlocillin is the most effective of the ureidopenicillins and superior to the carbenicillins (Wise et al, 1978).

Piperacillin has a fairly high incidence of allergic reactions.

Ceftazidime is the best of the new cephalosporins (Heilesen et al, 1983). It is expensive, but probably the most potent anti-pseudomonal agent developed to date. We reserve it for patients who are known to be allergic to penicillin (bearing in mind the five per cent cross-sensitivity with the cephalosporins) and for those who have shown an inadequate response to other agents.

Dosage and mode of administration

This is important. *CF patients require high doses of most antibiotics, because of inefficient penetration into sputum and increased renal clearance* (Kelly et al, 1982). In the presence of normal renal function (which is usual in CF) gentamicin and tobramycin should be given in doses of at least 2.5mg/kg/8 hours for children (Table IV) and serum levels monitored at 48 hours. 'Peak' levels, taken at 10 minutes after bolus short, or after a 30 minute infusion, should be at least 8mg/L (not more than 12mg/L) and 'trough'levels (which correlate better with the side effects of ototoxicity and nephrotoxicity) should be less than 2.0mg/L. Duration of treatment should be at least 10 days, but courses of two, three or even four weeks may be appropriate if respiratory function continues to improve.

Administration is usually by *bolus shot* for the aminoglycosides (this can be irritant and small infusions are necessary for some patients) and *by infusion,* well diluted, for the penicillins and cephalosporins. These drugs may be given consecutively, but not mixed together. Some of the penicillins, in particular, can be very irritant to peripheral veins. A 'Venflon' catheter with a 'Hepsal' (heparin-saline) lock is usually satisfactory for several days, sometimes a week, and allows the patient mobility and independence from the drip stand. This system may also be used at home.

It is sometimes difficult to assess, at the end of a course of treatment, whether the antibiotics or the expert physiotherapy has been of predominant benefit; they complement each other (Beaudry et al, 1980).

Antibiotics may also be given by inhalation. For control of pseudomonas infection, either colistin or a combination of gentamicin and carbenicillin are useful, although they will not eradicate the organism (see page 69).

TREATMENT BY INHALATION THERAPY

This may be used as an adjunct to treatment, both in hospital and at home, for periods of several months or in the longer term.

Efficacy is not easy to evaluate but many studies have shown its benefit (e.g. Hodson, Penketh and Batten, 1981; Heaf, Webb and Matthew, 1983). Improvement in survival rates, in one clinic, have been related to the introduction of aerosol antibiotics (Anderson, 1967 and Figure 16) although this interpretation has been challenged (Phelan and Hey, 1984).

Experiments with isotope-labelled aerosols have indicated that only 6–10 per cent of nebulized material actually reaches the lungs. Particle size should be five microns or less.

Mode of administration

The substance to be 'nebulized' is converted into a mist, by passing an air stream through it, and this is delivered to the patient via a face mask or mouth-piece. The air-stream is produced either by an electric motor, so that the nebulizer and motor form one portable unit (Figure 16) or the nebulizer can be driven by oxygen or air, at 4–6L/min, from a piped supply in hospital or from cylinders.

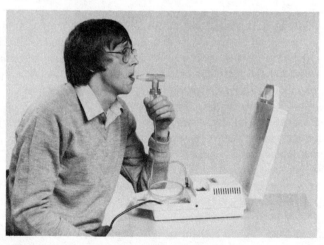

Figure 16. CF patient using portable nebulizer unit. Note that the nebulizer itself (held in the hand) is very close to the mouth piece

TABLE V. Examples of agents which may be given by aerosol

Agent	Volume or concentration	Comment
Moisturiser 0.9% saline	3ml	Liquefies mucus. Give *before* physiotherapy
Mucolytic agent Acetylcysteine	3ml of 20% solution. Can be diluted to 10% with saline	Liquifies mucus. May be irritant, avoid after haemoptysis
Bronchodilators Salbutamol (Ventolin) respirator solution	0.5ml (2.5mg) + 2.5ml normal (0.9%) saline	Bronchodilator. Give *before* physiotherapy
Terbutaline (Bricanyl) respirator solution	1.0ml (2.5mg) + 2.5ml normal (0.9%) saline	Bronchodilator. CF patients may note less tachycardia than with Salbutamol
Antibiotics Colistin sulphomethate sodium (Colomycin) ('Polymixin E')	250,000–1,000,000 units suspended in 2–4ml normal saline	Antipseudomonas, poorly absorbed systemically. Give antibiotic inhalations *after* physiotherapy
Gentamicin	20–80mg	each suspended in 2–4ml normal saline	Antipseudomonas and broad spectrum. Give consecutively
Carbenicillin	250mg – 1g		Carbenicillin has unpleasant smell – better used *before* gentamicin

Inhalations are usually given twice daily, dosage according to age

Ultrasonic nebulizers are also available, which give an even smaller particle size, but these are expensive and more difficult to maintain.

Volumes of mixtures for inhalation are 2—4ml and inhalations are given once, twice or three times daily — usually twice.

Types of inhalation

Examples of aerosols which may be given are shown in Table V.

Care of inhalation apparatus

Components of the nebulizer itself, and the tubing, should be cleaned thoroughly daily using a liquid detergent and clear running water — otherwise the machine will become blocked with sticky deposits and each treatment will take longer than the usual 10—15 minutes.

Mist tent therapy

Some years ago, nebulizers were employed to produce a fine water mist which was blown into a plastic tent in which the patient slept at night. However, studies have shown that these tents did not improve pulmonary function and may have encouraged the growth of pseudomonas. Many patients and parents disliked them. Their use has now been abandoned.

FUNGAL INFECTIONS

Invasive fungal infections are rare, although precipitins to aspergillus are often found.

Allergic aspergillosis should be suspected in any CF patient with marked bronchospasm. Relevant investigations are eosinophil count, skin tests (types I and III), measurement of IgE and RAST, precipitins and examination of the sputum for fungi (visualisation of hyphae and culture). Any one or most of these may be negative. When the diagnosis is truly positive, a good or even dramatic response may be obtained by treatment with corticosteroids (Brueton et al, 1980). Rare, unresponsive patients may require a specific antifungal agent in addition — intravenous miconazole or amphotericin. Oral ketoconazole, initially promising, should be used with caution in CF patients, in view of recent reports of cholestatic liver damage and androgen blocking activity (Hay, 1985).

The occasional patient with pneumonia due to invasive mycotic infection will also require systemic treatment with amphotericin.

Colonization of sputum with *Candida albicans* is not uncommon, but often transient. If serious candida pneumonia occurs, oral 5-fluorocytosine is effective (Jenner, Landau and Phelan, 1979).

VIRAL INFECTIONS

These may predispose to bacterial infections or even act synergistically with *Pseudomonas aeruginosa* (Petersen, Hoiby and Mordhorst, 1981). Wang et al (1984) conducted a comprehensive study of viral infection among CF patients and found significant correlations between the annual incidence of viral infection and every measure of disease progression over a two-year period.

Vaccination against influenza is probably worthwhile (see page 49).

RESPIRATORY COMPLICATIONS

Upper respiratory tract

Polyps A nasal spray, beclomethasone dipropionate (Beconase) may be tried when obstruction is incomplete. The unusual situation of complete obstruction may warrant polypectomy but repeated operations may be necessary.

Sinusitis Only a few patients have acute sinusitis, although X-rays will reveal mucosal thickening or opacity in the majority of older patients. Sinus washouts are rarely beneficial and never indicated on the basis of X-ray findings alone.

Otitis media There may be an increased incidence, associated with an obstruction of the Eustachian tubes, producing a conductive hearing loss.

High frequency hearing loss may be encountered with the aminoglycosides, but this seems unusual. *This was not the case, however, when neomycin was given by inhalation* and its use has been largely abandoned.

Lower respiratory tract

Viscous mucus Mucolytic agents may be useful. These can be by *inhalation* (Table V) or *orally* e.g. bromhexine hydrochloride (Bisolvon) carbocysteine (Mucodyne) or acetylcysteine (Fabrol). There is little evidence of the long-term value of oral agents. Their effect is said not to be optimal for several days. Epigastric pain is a side effect reported occasionally (presumably due to thinning of gastrointestinal mucus), and is a reason to withdraw treatment.

Cough Generally cough suppressants should be avoided. Clearance of respiratory mucus is the primary aim.

Bronchospasm This occurs sometimes, particularly in younger patients (less than 5 years) and in association with infection. Nebulized bronchodilators may be useful (Table V) as may inhalers: beta$_2$ stimulants, e.g. salbutamol (Ventolin) or anticholinergic agents, e.g. ipratropium bromide (Atrovent). Measurement of respiratory function before and after treatment will show whether these inhalers are really worthwhile for a particular patient.

Prophylaxis of true asthma (sometimes coexistent with CF) may be achieved with sodium cromoglycate (Intal). Long-term treatment may involve corticosteroid inhalers (i.e. beclomethasone dipropionate (Becotide), budesonide (Pulmicort) or corticosteroids by mouth.

There is no established indication for the use of corticosteroids in CF apart from coexistent asthma and allergic aspergillosis (see page 70).

Pneumothorax This becomes more common in the older patient. Many episodes will subside spontaneously, but intercostal drainage with insertion of a tube, or surgical intervention may be necessary (Penketh et al, 1982).

Haemoptyses Small streaks of blood occur quite often and the patient should be reassured. Larger bleeds, aggravated in some cases by abnormalities of coagulation, may happen in those with more serious lung disease. Treatment includes: bed rest, some reduction of physiotherapy, vitamin K by injection and transfusion. Persistent and severe bleeds may be checked by bronchial artery catheterization (to localize the site of bleeding) and embolization, using gelatin foam, to block off the point of bleeding (Figure 17) (Fellows, Khaw and Schuster, 1979). This is a specialized technique, available at a few centres only.

Localized atelectasis On occasions, a collapsed lobe or lung may be resistant to medical treatment, but may reinflate following *bronchoscopy and suction* to remove purulent secretions.

Figure 17. Series of X-rays to show bronchial artery catheterization
and embolization
(These pictures are by courtesy of Dr. M Ruttley, Department of Radiology,
University Hospital of Wales, Cardiff)

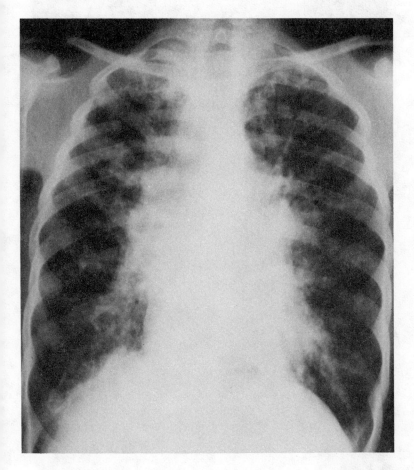

(a) Chest X-ray before the procedure, showing extensive bilateral disease. The
bleeding was coming from the right upper lobe

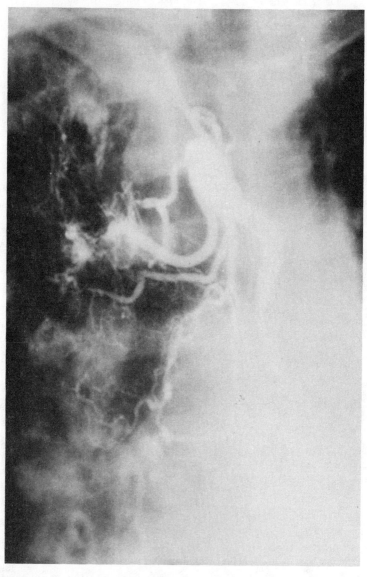

(b) Right bronchial arteriogram before embolization. Many leashes of blood
vessels are seen

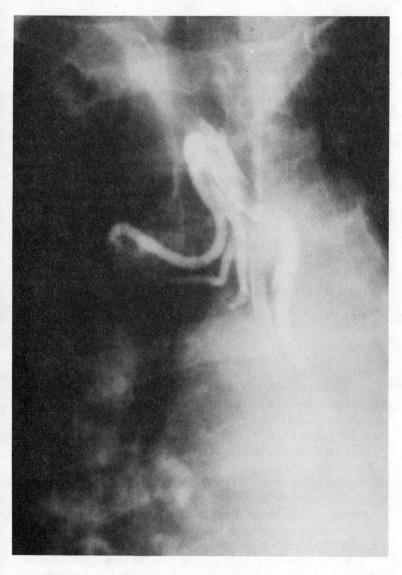

(c) After embolization with gelfoam and coil. The small blood vessels are now
occluded

Advanced respiratory disease

Pulmonary lavage Enthusiasm for this approach has varied. The procedure involves a general anaesthetic and actual lavage, via both main bronchi, using saline or other liquids. Post-operative management should be in an Intensive Care Unit with very frequent postural drainage and physiotherapy. Results have shown good short-term benefits (i.e. over several months) but long-term results are less clear. Some workers have advocated that lavage should be used *before* the onset of serious disease, but further studies are needed.

Pulmonary surgery This is rarely appropriate. Defined, segmental or lobar disease *may* be an indication, although lung pathology may be more widespread than some preoperative investigations would appear to indicate (i.e. radiology or isotope scans). A bronchogram should be done. Strenuous physiotherapy should be used together with other conservative measures for a long time, before considering surgery.

Tracheostomy or endotracheal intubation to permit mechanical ventilation is rarely used in the treatment of CF. It is an essential part of certain procedures (e.g. pulmonary lavage, see above) and it may be employed in a few, very ill patients for acute, potentially reversible lung disease.

Cor pulmonale

Progression of pulmonary disease inevitably results in the development of cor pulmonale, which is the most frequent cause of death in CF.

Right ventricular failure may occur suddenly during a severe flare-up of pulmonary disease or it may develop insidiously and become persistent. Clinical signs of cardiac failure are often difficult to detect, although cardiac dilatation, peripheral oedema and ascites may occur sometimes.

The severity of cor pulmonale appears to correlate quite well with arterial blood gas determinations and these may be valuable when deciding whether to institute treatment with diuretics or digoxin.

Diuretics should be used with caution both on account of their electrolyte-losing properties and their dehydrating action, which may exacerbate the dryness and stickiness of bronchial secretions.

The addition of digoxin can produce a further slight improvement, but again, serum electrolyte levels, particularly potassium levels, should be monitored.

Hypoxaemia

A paO_2 of less than 50mmHg is an indication for oxygen, either via a face mask or nasal spectacles. *However, many CF patients have chronic retention of CO_2 and depend on hypoxaemia for ventilatory drive.* Such patients should receive a low concentration of oxygen, 24–28 per cent, with measurement of blood gases.

Hypertrophic pulmonary osteoarthropathy (HPOA)

This curious, unusual complication is seen in many types of chronic chest disease, apart from CF. Typically, it affects older patients and larger joints i.e. knees and ankles. It is considered together with other joint problems which occasionally affect CF children, in chapter 7, page 123.

Air travel

This should present no problem, except for those with severe lung disease, who have a substantial reduction of arterial oxygen. Such patients should be advised not to travel unless controlled oxygen therapy can be provided on the aircraft.

PHYSIOTHERAPY

Adequate and consistent physiotherapy is probably the single most important factor in preventing chronic lung infection and in aiding antibiotics to eradicate infection.

It is vital for: (1) maintaining clear bronchial passages and ensuring adequate aeration of all parts of the lungs; (2) teaching correct patterns of breathing and effective coughing; (3) maintaining mobility of the chest wall and correct posture. It is important that it should be considered as a *preventive* as well as a *therapeutic* measure.

Physiotherapy should be started immediately after diagnosis and continued regularly each day, both during health and respiratory infection, when the numbers of treatments each day is usually increased.

Parents should be given a course of instruction by an experienced physiotherapist. This usually begins in hospital when the infant or child is first diagnosed, and the mother should be encouraged to live in the hospital for a few days, possibly longer, until she becomes proficient. It is very important to instruct the father also so that he can share the daily burden of therapy and involve himself in the child's care.

Refresher courses of instruction are also advisable at intervals during follow-up visits to the outpatient department especially as the child grows and different techniques become more suitable. Periodic visits to the home by a community physiotherapist are ideal if these can be

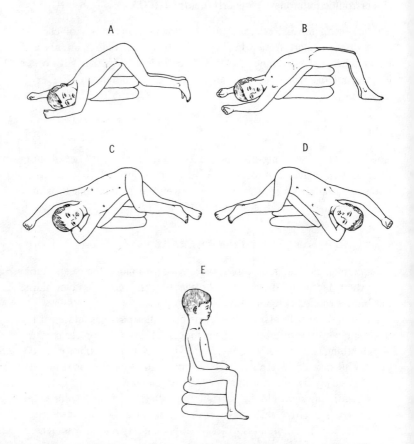

Figure 18. Illustration of positions used during physiotherapy for the chest in cystic fibrosis. The positions for draining the lower parts of the lungs are shown in A and B. The lateral parts of the lungs are drained in positions C and D, and the upper parts in position E

arranged. As the patient approaches adolescence, problems may occur in maintaining the treatment and at this time especially, the skills of a community physiotherapist can be invaluable.

Main features of technique

The aim is to loosen sputum in all areas of the lung and to encourage the patient to expel these secretions by coughing. Treatment is carried out in several different positions, having regard to the direction of optimal drainage of the individual lobes of the lungs. Techniques vary according to the age of the patient.

The infant and young child is placed in *five basic positions* either on the parent's lap or on a pile of cushions (Figure 18). *Percussion* of the chest, using cupped hands, is performed in each of the five positions, for about three minutes in each position, so that the total time for physiotherapy is 15–20 minutes. *Vibrations* and *rib-springing,* over a minute or so in each position, may be helpful also.

The older child may be treated in the same way, over a cushion (Figure 19) or, he/she may be taught a different, but equally effective technique, termed *forced expiration technique or FET.*

Forced expiration technique (FET)

This technique can be performed by the patient by himself, without the assistance of another person. It involves taking a *medium* inspiration (not a deep one) and then giving a forced and slightly prolonged expiration. This forced expiration, or *huff,* is frequently followed by coughing and the expiration of more sputum than can be achieved by simple coughing alone. Gentle diaphragmatic breathing alternates with one or two huffs.

Chest compression using the patient's own flexed arm (Figure 20) or help from an assistant, may be combined with FET, to increase sputum production.

FET may be used in isolation as a method of clearing sputum. However it can be used also in conjunction with percussion in postural drainage positions (Figure 20).

Thus FET can be ideal for the adolescent and adult patient particularly if he is living away from home in lodgings or at university.

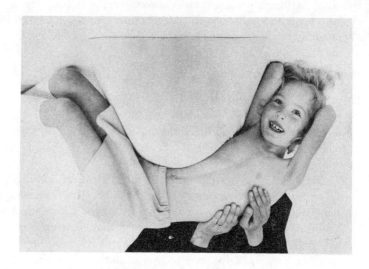

Figure 19. Sorbo-rubber pillow used for chest physiotherapy at home

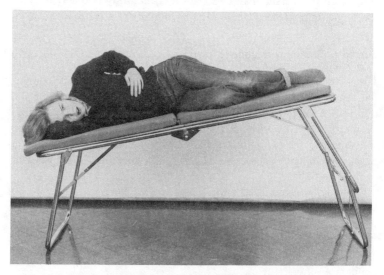

Figure 20. Same patient as shown in Figure 19, 10 years later, performing forced
   expiration technique (FET) and incorporating chest compression with her own
   flexed arm. She is lying on a Chesham Postural Drainage Frame

Additional points relating to physiotherapy are as below.

(1)   *The most effective time for physiotherapy is in the early morning, before breakfast,* so that secretions that have accumulated during the night can be expelled.

(2)   Treatments may be once, twice, or three or more times daily, depending on need.

(3)   Physiotherapy should be *before meals* and the occasional baby who may vomit, should be given extra feeds to compensate for lost calories.

(4)   While conventional physiotherapy is regarded as the principal method of clearing the lungs, it is increasingly realised that *exercise* and *games,* e.g. swimming, running, netball, dancing etc can make an important contribution to good health, and are probably more enjoyable. However, if exercise is used in place of physiotherapy it should be carried out on a regular, daily basis and not sporadically. A good compromise is one session of physiotherapy, and one of exercise, each day.
Trampolines may be effective in young children.

(5)   Hand-held mechanical *percussors* have been developed over the last few years but there is no evidence that these are superior to the efforts of the patient himself, or those of an assistant.

REFERENCES AND GENERAL READING

General

Andersen DH. Pathological anatomy of the early changes. In McIntosh R, ed. *Research on Cystic Fibrosis: Transactions of the 2nd International Research Conference on Cystic Fibrosis.* Bethesda, Ma, USA: NIAMD, 1960: 19–23

Anderson CM. Long-term study of patients with cystic fibrosis. *Bibl Paediatr 1967; 86:* 344–349

Beardsmore CS, Godfrey S, Katznelson D. Lung function in infants with cystic fibrosis. In *Proceedings of 12th Annual Meeting, EWGCF, Athens, Greece.* Athens: S Lennis. 1983: 11–15

Evans KT, Roberts GM. The chest radiograph in cystic fibrosis. *X-ray Focus 1978; 16 (3):* 62–73

Godfrey S, Mearns MB, Howlett G. Serial lung function tests in cystic fibrosis in the first 5 years of life. *Arch Dis Childh 1978; 53:* 83–85

Lloyd-Still JD, Khaw K-T, Shwachman H. Severe respiratory disease in infants with cystic fibrosis. *Pediatrics 1974; 53:* 678–682

Ormerod LP, Thomson RA, Anderson CM et al. Reversible airway obstruction in cystic fibrosis. *Thorax 1980; 35:* 768–771

Phelan P, Hey E. Cystic fibrosis mortality in England and Wales and in Victoria, Australia 1976–1980. *Arch Dis Childh 1984; 59:* 71–73

Taylor B, Evans JNG, Hope GA. Upper respiratory tract in cystic fibrosis, ear, nose and throat survey of 50 children. *Arch Dis Childh 1974; 49:* 133–136

Wilmott RW, Tyson SL, Dinwiddie R et al. Survival rates in cystic fibrosis. *Arch Dis Childh 1983; 58:* 835–836

Bacteriology, mycology, virology etc

Bergan T. Pathogenetic factors of Pseudomonas aeruginosa. *Scand J Infect Dis 1981; Suppl 29:* 7–12

Brueton MJ, Ormerod CP, Shah KJ et al. Allergic bronchopulmonary aspergillosis complicating cystic fibrosis in childhood. *Arch Dis Childh 1980; 55:* 348–353

Burns MW, May JR. Bacterial precipitins in serum of patients with cystic fibrosis. *Lancet 1968; i:* 270–272

Editorial. Anonymous. Cystic fibrosis and Pseudomonas infection. *Lancet 1983; ii:* 257–258

Hay RJ. Ketoconazole: a reappraisal. *Br Med J 1985; 1:* 260–261

Hoiby N. Microbiology of lung infections in cystic fibrosis patients. *Acta Paediatr Scand 1982; Suppl 301:* 33–54

Hoiby N, Friis B, Jensen K et al. Antimicrobial chemotherapy in cystic fibrosis patients. *Acta Paediatr Scand 1982; Suppl 301:* 75–100

Hoiby N, Schiotz PO. Immune complex mediated tissue damage in the lungs of cystic fibrosis patients with chronic Pseudomonas aeruginosa infection. *Acta Paediatr Scand 1982; Suppl 301:* 63–73

Isles A, Maclusky I, Corey M et al. Pseudomonas cepacia infection in cystic fibrosis: an emerging problem. *J Pediatr 1984; 104:* 206–210

Jenner BM, Landau LI, Phelan PD. Pulmonary candidiasis in cystic fibrosis. *Arch Dis Childh 1979; 54:* 555–556

Kulczycki LL, Murphy TM, Bellanti JA. Pseudomonas colonization in cystic fibrosis. *JAMA 1978; 240:* 30–34

Kulczycki LL, Wientzen RL, Bellanti JA et al. Why are some cystic fibrosis patients free of Pseudomonas colonization? In *Cystic Fibrosis: Horizons. Proceedings of the 9th International CF Congress, Brighton, England.* Chichester: John Wiley and Sons. 1984

Langford D, Hiller J. A prospective, controlled study of a polyvalent Pseudomonas vaccine in patients with cystic fibrosis. *Proceedings of the 12th Annual Meeting European Working Group for Cystic Fibrosis, Athens, Greece.* Athens: S Lennis. 1983

Lawson D, Porter T. Serum precipitins against respiratory tract pathogens in normal children and cystic fibrosis patients treated with cloxacillin. *Arch Dis Childh 1976; 51:* 890–891

Macone AB, Pier GB, Pennington JE et al. Mucoid Escherichia coli in cystic fibrosis. *N Engl J Med 1981; 304:* 1445–1449

May JR, Herrick WC, Thompson D. Bacterial infection in cystic fibrosis. *Arch Dis Childh 1972; 47:* 908–913

McCrae WM, Raeburn JA. Patterns of infection in cystic fibrosis. *Scot Med J 1974; 19:* 187–190

Mearns MB. Natural history of pulmonary infection in cystic fibrosis. In *Perspectives in Cystic Fibrosis. Proceedings of the 8th International CF Congress, Toronto, Canada*. Ontario: Canadian CF Foundation. 1980: 325–334

Mearns MB, Hunt GH, Rushworth R. Bacterial flora of respiratory tract in patients with cystic fibrosis. *Arch Dis Childh 1972; 47:* 902–907

Petersen NT, Hoiby N, Mordhorst CH. Respiratory infections in cystic fibrosis patients caused by virus, chlamydia and mycoplasma – possible synergism with Pseudomonas aeruginosa. *Acta Paediatr Scand 1981; 70:* 623–628

Reynolds HY, di Sand'Agnese PA, Zierdt CH. Mucoid Pseudomonas aeruginosa: a sign of cystic fibrosis in young adults with chronic pulmonary disease? *JAMA 1976: 236:* 2190–2192

Wang EEL, Prober CG, Manson B et al. Association of respiratory viral infections with pulmonary deterioration in patients with cystic fibrosis. *N Engl J Med 1984; 311:* 1653–1658

Zierdt CH, Schmidt PJ. Dissociation in Pseudomonas aeruginosa. *J Bacteriol 1964; 87:* 1003

Antibiotic and aerosol treatment

Beaudry PH, Marks MI, McDougall et al. Is anti-Pseudomonas therapy warranted in acute respiratory exacerbations in children with cystic fibrosis? *J Pediatr 1980; 97:* 144–151

Editorial. Anonymous. The quinolones. *Lancet 1984; i:* 24–25

Heaf DP, Webb GJ, Matthew DJ. In vitro assessment of combined antibiotic and mucolytic treatment of Pseudomonas aeruginosa infection in cystic fibrosis. *Arch Dis Childh 1983; 58:* 824–826

Heilesen AM, Permin H, Koch C et al. Treatment of chronic Pseudomonas aeruginosa infection in cystic fibrosis patients with ceftazidime and tobramycin. *Scand J Infec Dis 1983; 15:* 271–276

Hodson ME, Penketh ARL, Batten JC. Aerosol carbenicillin and gentamicin treatment of Pseudomonas aeruginosa infections in patients with cystic fibrosis. *Lancet 1981; ii:* 1137–1139

Hodson ME, Wingfield HJ, Batten JC. Tobramycin and carbenicillin compared with gentamicin and carbenicillin in the treatment of infection with Pseudomonas aeruginosa in adult patients with cystic fibrosis. *Br J Dis Chest 1983; 77:* 71–77

Huang NN, Harley RD, Promadhattavedi V et al. Visual disturbances in cystic fibrosis following chloramphenicol administration. *J Pediat 1966; 68:* 32–44

Kelly HB, Menendez R, Fan L et al. Pharmacokinetics of tobramycin in cystic fibrosis. *J Pediatr 1982; 100:* 318–321

Knight RJ. Antibiotic doses for the bronchiectasis of cystic fibrosis. *Lancet 1983; ii:* 970–971 (letter)

Lerner AM, Reyes MP, Cone LA et al. Randomised, controlled trial of the comparative efficacy, auditory toxicity and nephrotoxicity of Tobramycin and Netilmicin. *Lancet 1983; i:* 1123–1126

Phelan PD, Gracey M, Williams HE et al. Ventilatory function in infants with cystic fibrosis: physiological assessment of inhalation therapy. *Arch Dis Childh 1969; 44:* 393–400

Smith CR, Lipsky JJ, Laskin OL et al. Double-blind comparison of the nephrotoxicity and auditory toxicity of gentamicin and tobramycin. *N Engl J Med 1980; 302:* 1106–1109

Szaff M, Hoiby N, Flensborg EW. Frequent antibiotic therapy improves survival of cystic fibrosis patients with chronic Pseudomonas aeruginosa infection. *Acta Paediatr Scand 1983; 72:* 651–657

Winter RJD, George RJD, Deacock SJ et al. Self-administered home intravenous antibiotic therapy in bronchiectasis and adult cystic fibrosis. *Lancet 1984; i:* 1338–1339

Wise R, Gillett AP, Andrews JM et al. Activity of Azlocillin and Mezlocillin against gram-negative organisms: comparison with other penicillins. *Antimicrob Agents and Chemotherapy 1978; 13:* 559–565

Respiratory complications

Fellows KE, Khaw K-T, Schuster S. Bronchial artery embolization in cystic fibrosis: technique and long-term results. *J Pediatr 1979; 95:* 959–963

Kulczycki LL. Experience with 632 bronchoscopic bronchial washings done on 173 cystic fibrosis patients during a 16 year period (1965–1980).
In Warwick WJ, ed. *1000 Years of Cystic Fibrosis.* Minnesota: University of Minnesota. 1981: 95–112

Mearns MB, Hodson CJ, Jackson ADM et al. Pulmonary resection in cystic fibrosis. Results in 23 cases, 1957–70. *Arch Dis Childh 1972; 47:* 499–508

Penketh ARL, Knight RK, Hodson ME et al. Management of pneumothorax in adults with cystic fibrosis. *Thorax 1982; 37:* 850–853

Whitman V, Stern RC, Bellet P et al. Studies on cor pulmonale in cystic fibrosis.
1. Effects of diuresis. *Pediatrics 1975; 55:* 83–85

Physiotherapy

Gaskell DV, Webber B. *The Physical Treatment of Cystic Fibrosis.* Bromley, Kent, England: Cystic Fibrosis Research Trust. 1982

Geddes DM. Physical exercise and cystic fibrosis. In *Cystic Fibrosis: Horizons. Proceedings of the 9th International CF Congress, Brighton, England.* Chichester: John Wiley & Sons. 1984: 117–138

Maxwell M. Review of literature of physiotherapy in cystic fibrosis. *Physiotherapy 1980; 66:* 245–246

Maxwell M, Redmond A. Comparative trial of manual and mechanical percussion technique with gravity-assisted bronchial drainage in patients with cystic fibrosis. *Arch Dis Childh 1979; 54:* 542–544

Pryor JA, Webber BA, Hodson ME et al. Evaluation of the forced expiration technique as an adjunct to postural drainage in treatment of cystic fibrosis. *Br Med J 1979; 2:* 417–418

Weller PH, Bush E, Preece MA et al. Short-term effects of chest physiotherapy on pulmonary function in children with cystic fibrosis. *Respiration 1980; 40:* 53–56

Zach M, Oberwaldner B, Hausler F. Cystic fibrosis: physical exercise versus chest physiotherapy. *Arch Dis Childh 1982; 57:* 587–589

Reviews

Campbell IA, Schonell M. *Respiratory Medicine: 2nd Edn.* Edinburgh: Churchill Livingstone. 1984

Marks MI. The pathogenesis and treatment of pulmonary infections in patients with cystic fibrosis. *J Pediatr 1981: 98:* 173–179

Mearns MB. Personal practice. Cystic fibrosis. *Arch Dis Childh 1985; 60:* 272–277

Moss RB. Immunology of cystic fibrosis: immunity, immunodeficiency and hypersensitivity. In Lloyd-Still JD, ed. *Textbook of Cystic Fibrosis.* Bristol: John Wright. 1983: 109–151

Nielsen OH, Schiotz PO. Cystic fibrosis in Denmark in the period 1945–1981. Evaluation of centralized treatment. *Acta Paediatr Scand 1982; suppl 301:* 107–119

Chapter 6

MANAGEMENT OF NUTRITIONAL PROBLEMS

At least three major factors are responsible for the nutritional problems which often arise in cystic fibrosis. These are:

1. malabsorption resulting mainly from pancreatic insufficiency;

2. chronic respiratory infection (and later hypoxia);

3. poor nutritional intake.

There is also some evidence that the *intrinsic requirement for calories is raised in CF* (i.e. there is an increased basal metabolic rate).

The majority of CF patients have pancreatic enzyme insufficiency, with low concentrations of digestive enzymes in the small gut, from birth; in a small minority this develops later (see Chapter 2). Enzymes affected include amylase, trypsin and lipase, which are important for the digestion of carbohydrate, protein and fat, respectively. In addition, the absorption of fat-soluble vitamins, A,E,K and possibly D, is also impaired.

In older patients, especially, *there may be a reduction in the amount of bile salts secreted into the duodenum.* Bile salts have a detergent effect, helping to emulsify fats and make them available for the action of lipase — whether produced from the pancreas or taken as a supplement. The effect of bile salt production on digestion of fats is therefore additional to that of pancreatic enzyme insufficiency.

Malabsorption results in offensive, abnormally bulky and frequent stools, containing undigested fat and protein. In addition to the loss of calories, such stools have a penetrating, 'cheesy' odour which is a source of embarrassment to the patient and is a further reason for minimising malabsorption.

Uncontrolled respiratory infection is another important cause of a poor gain in weight. The degree of malnutrition corresponds more closely to the severity of respiratory involvement than to the malabsorption (Lapey et al, 1974; Kraemer et al, 1978).

Although infants with CF usually have a ravenous appetite, older children and adults, particularly those with significant chest disease, often eat less than their recommended daily allowance of calories — average total food intakes of approximately 80 per cent of the recommended daily allowance have been recorded (Chase, Long and Lavin, 1979). Theoretical calculations suggest that in order to compensate for the excess calories lost in the stools (even when pancreatic supplements are given) and the increased calorie requirements which are especially marked in the presence of chronic infection, an intake of about 150 per cent of the recommended daily allowance is necessary (Shwachman, 1978; Dodge, 1985). This can rarely be achieved in advanced respiratory disease unless special nutritional supplements are given.

ASSESSMENT OF NUTRITION

Essential data include measurements of **growth** and calculation of **dietary intake**.

Growth

From the time of diagnosis until growth is complete, serial measurements should be made of weight and height and when appropriate, head circumference and skinfold thickness.

Slowing of growth velocity or actual weight loss is an indication that something is amiss. These are some of the most sensitive indices of chest infection, sometimes occurring *even before* the patient or parents complain of any worsening of symptoms. We consider that frequent weighing is as important as regular lung function testing (which in any case is difficult to carry out in the very young child, without complex equipment).

Measurements of growth (weight and height) should be plotted on standard growth charts appropriate to the child's race — charts for British children are shown in modified form in Figure 21a and b. *Centile lines* on these charts (e.g. 3rd, 50th, 97th) record the increase in weight

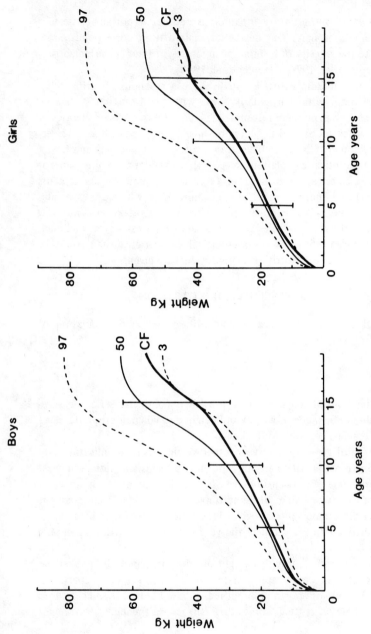

Figure 21a. Weight centile charts for boys and girls with cystic fibrosis, aged 0–19 years. (For explanation of centile lines 3, 50 and 97, see text). Dark lines (CF) show median weight gain for CF patients; the vertical bars indicate ranges of weights for these patients at 5, 10 and 15 years

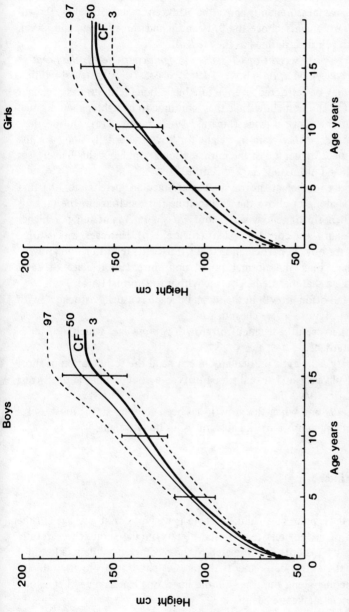

Figure 21b. Height centile charts, drawn in a similar fashion to Figure 21a. Dark lines (CF) show median height gain for CF patients, the vertical bars the ranges of heights for these patients at 5, 10 and 15 years. These charts (21a and b) have been redrawn from Mearns MB. In Hodson ME, Norman AP, Batten JC, eds. *Cystic Fibrosis 1983*, with permission

or height for defined sections of the population. Out of 100 children, 50 will have measurements above the 50th centile and 50 below; 97 will have measurements above the 3rd centile and three below, and so on. The 50th centile is defined as the *median.*

Average birth-weight of CF babies is significantly lower than that of the normal population (Boyer, 1955; Yassa, 1979) suggesting that growth may be restricted, even before birth. Long-term studies of weight gain in CF children show that they continue to be lighter than normal, although the range is wide (Mearns, 1983, Figure 21a). During their first decade, *median* gain in weight for boys and girls is along, or just below, the 25th centile of the normal population; later, this line crosses the 10th and ultimately the 3rd centile.

Records for height are rather better: median increase for the first decade is along or above the 25th centile (although again, the range is wide) then shifting downwards but in general maintaining a higher centile than the record for weight (Figure 21b). However, a reassuring feature, for boys in particular, is that CF patients tend to go on growing for longer than the normal population, into late teenage or early twenties, so that mature heights are within the normal range.

The fall-off in growth in the second decade is usually associated with the onset of more severe chest disease.

Another useful assessment of growth is *bone age* which also tends to be retarded.

Puberty is delayed particularly in *boys* and the combination of short stature, physical and sexual immaturity is a common cause of distress to teenagers.

In *adults* and when the growth has been completed, the most useful check of a patient's nutritional status is his body weight.

Dietary intake

If growth is poor in a child, or there is weight loss at any age (in the absence of an obvious reason) the dietary intake should be carefully checked by a dietitian and related to the recommended daily allowance and to the extra requirements of the CF patient. If growth velocity is proceeding along the usual centile lines, one can assume that calorie and protein intake are adequate.

DIETARY MANAGEMENT

General principles

1. *Dietary manipulations should be kept to a minimum.* Children with CF suffer considerable inconvenience because of their multiple treatments and it is unwise to impose further problems by dietary restrictions which do not have any proven long-term benefit. It is more important that parents continue to carry out treatments aimed at keeping the chest infection under control, rather than to waste time preparing food different from that of the rest of the family. Dietary restrictions make the child feel different at school and among friends.

   The majority of CF children who do not have serious chest symptoms and who are taking adequate pancreatic supplements, are able to take a normal diet without difficulty.

2. The meals, however, should be increased in *quantity* for the CF person, and have a *high protein high calorie* and usually a *normal fat* content. Starchy foods should not be given in excess, but disaccharides and monosaccharides are well utilized.

   When CF children are well they will often eat as much as adults and enjoy second helpings and snacks.

   The required calorie intake for CF children, including babies, is frequently considerably greater than for normal children.

3. *In general, a normal, or near normal amount of fat can be tolerated* provided that pancreatic supplements are sufficient to assist with its digestion. The development of more effective preparations of pancreatic enzymes (see page 92) has been helpful in allowing a more liberal fat intake than has been the practice in the past. In some centres, high fat intakes have been encouraged (Crozier, 1974; MacDonald, 1984).

   Fat restriction may be required for some patients, but a very low fat diet is not only unappetising, but is likely to be low in calories, fat soluble vitamins and essential fatty acids (see page 100). For patients who are really intolerant of normal, long chain fat, e.g. meat fat, butter or margarine, substitution of some of this fat with *medium chain triglycerides* (oils and fat derived from coconut oil, page 99) may be helpful.

4. Some children fail to gain weight despite control of pulmonary infection and others show a progressive growth failure when pulmonary function deteriorates. Such patients need nutritional supplements taken with ordinary food, or special formulae (see page 101) to provide extra calories and protein.

5. *Special diets* are occasionally required for the few children who are *intolerant of lactose,* those who have *co-existent coeliac disease* or develop *diabetes mellitus.*

6. *Fat soluble vitamins* are poorly absorbed and should be supplemented. This applies particularly to vitamins A,D,E, and sometimes K.

A normal diet for CF children

The diet should include protein at least twice daily, e.g. lean meat, fish, eggs or cheese. Whole milk or skimmed milk are important constituents. Starchy food in excess may produce gaseous abdominal distension, discomfort and flatulence, but refined carbohydrates (sugars) are usually well absorbed.

The help of an experienced dietitian is invaluable and should be requested for all patients who are failing to thrive or who are losing weight.

PANCREATIC ENZYME REPLACEMENT

This is necessary for the majority of CF children but not for the 10 per cent or so who have residual pancreatic secretion. It is therefore important to examine the stools before treatment in order to document the presence of steatorrhoea.

Malabsorption may progress subsequently, even in those babies with good pancreatic function.

Pancreatic enzyme preparations (pancreatin)

These are usually derived from the hog and contain the enzymes trypsin, lipase and amylase. Some preparations also contain enzymes of plant origin and small amounts of bile salts, although the efficacy of these has yet to be determined.

Table VI lists some of the products; it is not exhaustive and not all are available in all countries.

There is a variety of presentations: powders; enteric coated granules; capsules containing powders or enteric coated granules; enteric coated tablets.

Powder is most suitable for infants and young children. It undergoes some inactivation in the stomach, due to acid gastric juice, but milk feeds have a considerable buffering action.

Enteric coating is designed to dissolve in an alkaline medium in the duodenum, but unfortunately, owing to defective bicarbonate production by the CF pancreas, compounded by increased acid production by the CF stomach (Cox, Isenberg and Ament, 1982) pH in the CF duodenum is rarely above neutral and a strong enteric coating may not be penetrated. *Enteric coated granules (e.g. Creon, Pancrease)* are the most satisfactory preparations even from the toddler age group, and give the best values for protein and fat absorption (Gow et al, 1981).

Unless protected by a coating of some kind, pancreatin is not pleasant to take.

Mode of administration

Pancreatic preparations should be taken just before, or during the meal, and with each meal. A further allowance should be given with between-meal snacks if these contain milk or foods other than fruit.

Powder for infants and young children may be mixed with a little milk (cow's milk, formula milk or even breast milk) or food on a teaspoon. Fresh powder (from the container or capsule) should be used with each feed. *It should not be mixed with the milk in the feeding bottle* as it will curdle the milk so blocking the teat, *nor sprinkled onto the meal itself as it makes the food unpalatable.*

Tablets for older children or adults are more effective if they are chewed although this releases the tangy taste.

Enteric coated granules are both more acceptable and more effective. The granules should not be chewed. The gelatin capsule in which they are presented dissolves readily in most patients and it is probably not necessary to remove the granules from the capsule before use.

Dosage

This is individual and there is a wide range. Guidelines are given in Table VI. An adequate dose is one which reduces the size, frequency

TABLE VI. Pancreatic enzyme preparations

A) Preparations (listed alphabetically) available as capsules (containing powder) and enteric coated tablets

Preparation	Presentation	Dose (Doses are for guidance only. Vary according to clinical symptoms)	Comments
Cotazyme (Organon Laboratories Ltd)	Capsules	*Up to 6–9 months*: contents of. ½–1 capsule per feed. *For older children and adults*: 2–8 capsules with each meal, 1–2 with snacks	*Infants* can be given the powder (after opening the capsules) mixed with a little milk or yoghurt. *Older children and adults* swallow the capsules before and/or during the meal. *Do not sprinkle on the meal itself*
Cotazym B (Organon Laboratories Ltd)	Tablets	*For children and adults*: 2–8 tablets with each meal, 1–2 with snacks	Contain ox bile – do not chew as this releases the bitter taste
Nutrizym (E Merck Ltd)	Tablets	*For children and adults*: 2–8 tablets with each meal, 1 with snacks	External sugar coating. Bromelain shell and enteric coated core of pancreatin 400mg, ox bile 30mg
Pancrex V (Paines and Byrne Ltd)	Pancrex V capsules	*Up to 6–9 months*: contents of 1–2 capsules mixed with feeds. *Over 9 months*: contents of 2–6 capsules with each meal	Mix with a little milk, yoghurt, mashed potato, etc, give just before and/or during feed or meal. *Do not sprinkle onto the meal.* Used mainly for young children – older patients take tablets

(continued on next page)

Preparation	Presentation	Dose (Doses are for guidance only. Vary according to clinical symptoms)	Comments
	Pancrex V tablets	5–15 tablets with each meal, 1–2 with snacks	Tablets small and relatively tasteless. Suitable for younger children
	Pancrex V forte tablets	2–8 tablets with each meal, 1 with snacks	Larger tablets but contain approximately 3 times the enzyme dose of Pancrex V. Suitable for older children and adults

For table of comparative enzyme activities of various preparations, see British National Formulary

B) Enteric coated granule preparations

(These capsules, containing granules, are more recently formulated and more efficient, see page 93)

Preparation	Enzyme content per capsule (B.P. units)	Dose	Comments
Creon (Dulphar Laboratories Ltd)	Lipase 8000 Amylase 9000 Protease 210	*For young children:* contents of ½–1 capsule with each meal. *For older children and adults:* 1–4 capsules with each meal, 1 with snacks	If capsules opened (for young children) enteric coated granules may be mixed with a little food or drink, for ease of swallowing, *but should not be chewed* as this will destroy the enteric coating. The granules are tasteless unless chewed. Capsules may be swallowed whole, before or during the meal.
Pancrease (Ortho-Cilag Pharmaceuticals Ltd U.K, McNeil Laboratories, USA)	Lipase 5000 Amylase 3000 Protease 350	*For young children:* contents of 1–2 capsules with each meal. *For older children and adults:* 2–5 capsules with each meal, 1 with snacks	

and consistency of stools to the optimum for that patient, and ensures that the child thrives (provided that chest infection and other problems are under control).

Generally, dosage should not be altered more often than every few days or once a week in order to make the best assessment.

Strenuous efforts to achieve completely normal stools are usually unrewarding: steatorrhoea is rarely eliminated but can be very considerably reduced. *Percentage fat absorption* should be expected to rise from an average baseline of about 50 per cent (without pancreatic enzymes) to a minimum of 70 per cent and possibly to 85 per cent or more. This is still less than the figure of approximately 96 per cent which is found in normal persons (Goodchild et al, 1974; Gow et al,1981). *Snacks between meals should not be forgotten.* A common error is to raise the dose of pancreatin with main meals, if stools are abnormal, while forgetting the snacks.

There is little or no advantage in increasing dosages to very high levels. *If this appears to be necessary, the dietitian should prepare a detailed analysis of the child's intake and advise on fat reduction if this intake is excessive.* Alternatively, the effects of antacids and H_2-receptor antagonists (gastric acid suppressants) given in addition to pancreatic enzymes, may be tried.

Antacids and H_2-receptor antagonists

Pancreatic enzymes are most effective in an alkaline environment, which is often lacking in the CF duodenum (see above). Another approach therefore, is to give an antacid with the meal. Sodium bicarbonate in a high dosage ($15g/m^2/day$) is sometimes effective (Durie et al, 1980a). If it is tried, it may be given as 1.5g powder dissolved in half a glass of water, but results are variable and side-effects include abdominal distension and flatulence.

As a more acceptable alternative, agents which reduce gastric acid secretion, i.e. cimetidine (Tagamet) or ranitidine (Zantac) may be used. Several studies report an improvement in faecal fat and faecal nitrogen (Regan et al, 1979, Durie et al, 1980a). The long-term effects of these histamine receptor antagonists are not yet known, and their routine use is not advised in children. Short-term side-effects are few.

Side-effects of pancreatin

In young children, large doses may produce perioral and perianal irritation and some soreness, improved by barrier creams, but alleviated by dose reduction.

Occasional patients (and their parents) become allergic to hog pancreatin *in powder form,* developing asthma or skin rashes.

Abdominal pain and constipation is sometimes related to a high dose of pancreatin and is improved by reducing the dose. It is doubtful if this situation represents the 'meconium ileus equivalent' syndrome which is sometimes seen in older patients (Chapter 7).

Increased blood levels and urinary excretion of *uric acid* have been documented in patients taking very large doses of pancreatic extracts, but significant renal tubular damage has not been described (Davidson et al, 1978). These levels can drop to normal when pancreatic dosage is reduced.

BILE ACID METABOLISM

Several manoeuvres have been shown to curtail the excessive loss of faecal bile acids and so improve bile acid pool size (see Chapter 2, page 18). These include the use of pancreatic enzyme supplements (Weber et al, 1973; Watkins et al, 1977); the effect of cimetidine (which reduces the precipitation of bile acids within an acid environment) with pancreatic enzymes (Boyle et al, 1980; Zentler-Munro et al, 1981); replacement of some long chain fat by medium chain fat (MCT), taken with pancreatic enzymes (Smalley et al, 1978).

Bile salt additives or substitutes are not used at the moment as an effective and palatable formulation has yet to be prepared.

When liver disease is present it may be useful to substitute some long chain fat with MCT and provide adequate fat-soluble vitamin supplements.

VITAMINS AND OTHER SUPPLEMENTS

Vitamins

Clinically important deficiencies are confined to the fat-soluble vitamins A, E, K and occasionally D.

Vitamin A Levels are frequently reduced, despite the use of supplements. There is some evidence that storage and release from the liver is abnormal and serum levels of retinol-binding protein are also low. However, clinical signs of vitamin A deficiency are rare but have been the presenting feature of CF.

Vitamin D Curiously, rickets is extremely rare in CF. There is conflicting evidence on vitamin D absorption but it is probably slightly decreased in most patients. Total serum calcium levels are within the low-normal range (in the absence of hypoproteinaemia) but mineralization of bone may be poor.

Vitamin E Low concentrations are almost always present but the significance is unknown. Occasionally, in young infants, this causes a haemolytic anaemia and oedema, but no symptoms occur in the great majority of patients. Very severe and prolonged deficiency can give rise to neurological changes (Elias, Muller and Scott, 1981).

Vitamin K Deficiency (measured as a prolonged prothrombin time) produces impaired blood clotting and a tendency to excessive bleeding. Young infants with CF quite often show this problem, particularly those who have obstructive jaundice (prolonged neonatal jaundice) or who are breast-fed; it is also one of the first indices to become abnormal in patients who are developing overt liver disease. Vitamin K2 is synthesized by intestinal bacteria and this important secondary source is absent in neonates, and may be diminished at any age when broad spectrum antibiotics are given.

Dosage Vitamins should be given daily, or twice daily, in a total dosage of twice the normal recommended allowance for age and if possible, in water-soluble form.

None of the multivitamin products currently available contains sufficient *vitamin E* for CF requirements and it is generally considered that this should be given as a separate preparation, 200mg daily for adults and in water-soluble form. Fat-soluble vitamin E is not only poorly absorbed but seems to produce abdominal pain in some patients.

Vitamin K when necessary can be given orally and by injection. The oral vitamin should be the water-soluble variety, i.e. menadiol sodium diphosphate (Synkavit) and the dosage is 10mg daily for adults.

Mineral supplements

Iron Haemoglobin levels are usually well maintained but frank iron deficiency does occur sometimes. Even mild degrees of anaemia can be important in the presence of significant lung disease, when maximum oxygen carrying capacity by the blood is required. Standard iron supplements are usually well absorbed (Ater et al, 1983).

Zinc Low levels in plasma and erythrocytes have been reported in association with growth retardation (Neve et al, 1983). However, blood levels, hair levels and even white blood cell concentrations of zinc are unreliable indications of zinc status and there is no unequivocal evidence that zinc supplementation is appropriate in CF.

Selenium No convincing evidence has been put forward for the necessity or usefulness of selenium supplements in CF and selenium toxicity is quite easily induced, especially in the presence of vitamin E deficiency (Lloyd-Still and Ganther, 1980).

Medium chain triglycerides (MCT)

These oils and fats, mainly of chain length C8–C10, and derived from coconut oil, are absorbed more efficiently than long chain fats.

They may be used as dietary supplements to provide extra calories, or as partial replacement of the usual long chain dietary fat, when both steatorrhoea and faecal bile acid loss are reduced (Smalley et al, 1978; Durie et al, 1980b). Complete replacement of long chain fat is not desirable as this will induce a deficiency of essential fatty acids (see below).

Pancreatin supplements are required for optimal absorption (Durie et al, 1980b), as for the absorption of all fats in the treatment of cystic fibrosis.

MCT oil is a clear, straw-coloured liquid with a calorie value of 8.3Kcal/g oil (34.8kJ). It is a saturated fat, resistant to oxidation and does not go rancid in storage. It is normally almost tasteless but when used for cooking, for example for chips and fish, some practice is desirable to avoid overheating it, when it becomes bitter. It also has a low flash point and should not be left on a stove unattended.

The effects of MCT are not only to provide additional calories, but to reduce stool bulk, abdominal distension and discomfort.

Clinical situations in which MCT may be helpful include: malnutrition, particularly in infants recovering from meconium ileus and those who have had gut resection; steatorrhoea difficult to control by other means; recurrent rectal prolapse; chronic liver disease.

MCT products are available as the oil (Cow and Gate), incorporated into special milks, e.g. *Portagen, Pregestimil* (Bristol-Myers), see page 101, and as margarine (marketed in Germany and available in UK through hospitals only).

Essential fatty acids (EFA)

'Essential' fatty acids (EFA) cannot be manufactured within the body, so they must be taken in the food; nevertheless they are essential for certain metabolic purposes, including growth and production of cellular membranes; they are also precursors of prostaglandins.

Deficiency of EFA, particularly linoleic acid (18:2), has often been observed in CF. Theoretically, correction of EFA deficiency might be expected to produce clinical benefit but the studies reported to date have not been sufficiently impressive to justify routine EFA supplements (Rosenlund, Lim and Kritchevsky, 1974; Chase, Long and Lavin, 1979; Kussoffsky, Strandvik and Troell, 1983; Goodchild et al, 1984). When supplements of EFA are given, the requirement for vitamin E is further enhanced and additional vitamin E should also be prescribed.

INFANT FEEDING

The same principles apply to CF infants as to older children — their calorie intake should be increased, up to 150 per cent of the recommended dietary allowance; the majority will require pancreatin supplements with all milks even with breast-milk and formulae containing medium chain triglycerides (see page 99; vitamins should be given in water-miscible form, in twice the dosage recommended for non-CF infants, and vitamins E and K are usually included (Laing, 1985 and page 98).

Milks

Although a variety is available, many of them tailored to the needs of the CF child, we suggest that if breast-feeding is feasible, that "breast is best" for CF infants as for healthy newborns. *In addition to the better absorption of fat and protein from human milk compared to cow's milk formulae,* the mother who is coming to terms with the news that her baby has an inherited disease should have the satisfaction of knowing that she is contributing in a unique way to his care and providing the best possible nourishment.

If breast-feeding is not practicable or the mother does not wish to breast-feed, the CF baby may thrive perfectly well on standard, modified cow's milk formulae, e.g. gold cap SMA (Wyeth) or Premium (Cow and Gate). If not, a modified milk may be required, such as *Pregestimil* or *Nutramigen.*

Pregestimil (Bristol-Myers) or a similar preparation, is probably the milk of choice — protein is hydrolysed (partially digested), fat is a mixture of medium chain and long chain triglycerides and the carbohydrate is glucose.

Nutramigen (Bristol-Myers) is somewhat different — although the protein is hydrolysed, the fat is predominantly long chain and the carbohydrate is sucrose. However, Nutramigen is sometimes the more acceptable of the two milks, perhaps because of the better smell and taste.

Other 'milks' are quite suitable including *MCT Pepdite* 0–2 (Scientific Hospital Supplies) and a cheaper 'home-made' high protein/low fat mixture, as used in the Hospital for Sick Children, Great Ormond Street, London (Dinwiddie, 1983).

Supplements of glucose polymers such as *Caloreen* (Roussel) or *Maxijul* (Scientific Hospital Supplies) may be added to all milks.

At a practical level, *physiotherapy should be done before feeds,* with an interval between, and *the volume of any vomited feeds should be replaced.*

The baby recovering from meconium ileus often has special problems and may require full, intravenous parenteral nutrition. When oral feeds are resumed, the same general approach, with increased calorie intake and pancreatic enzyme supplements, applies.

NUTRITIONAL SUPPLEMENTATION

Simple, oral supplementation of normal diets for CF patients, with MCT products, glucose polymers, etc, has been in use for years with varying effectiveness.

TABLE VII. Examples of dietary supplements

Supplements	Use
Skimmed milk based powders	
1) Complan (Farley) Build-up (Carnation) and others	High protein powders which may be made up with milk (or water). Glucose powders and fat emulsion (see below) can be added in addition, to form a milk-shake. Available in several flavours
2) Commercially available skimmed milk powders	These may be added to cow's milk, yoghurts, etc, to increase protein and calorie content (as may ice-cream, raw eggs or Maxijul, see below)
High protein powders e.g. Maxipro HBV (Scientific Hospital Supplies) Casilan (Farley) *Glucose powders* e.g. Maxijul (Scientific Hospital Supplies) Caloreen (Roussel) Polycal (Cow and Gate)	May be added to foods or drinks (hot or cold), yoghurt
Fat emulsions e.g. Liquigen (Scientific Hospital Supplies) Calogen (Scientific Hospital Supplies) Prosparol (Duncan Flockhart)	May be added to foods and liquids, as above, but mix better with milk-based foods rather than with fruit-juices
Medium chain triglyceride oils e.g. Alembicol D (Alembic Products) MCT oil (Cow and Gate) MCT oil (Bristol Myers)	Used mainly in cooking and if fat tolerance is a problem. Absorption is improved with pancreatin supplements, see page 99

MISCELLANEOUS

Raw eggs can be quite palatable when added to milk, custards and fruit-juices.
Grated cheese can be mixed with mashed potato or sprinkled over soups or pasta.
Liquidized meats can be used to fortify soups.
Ice-cream can be added to milk

The 'Allan diet' (Allan, Mason and Moss, 1973) was an early attempt to provide an artificial, 'predigested' diet for CF patients. A comprehensive analysis of its use showed only marginal improvement in growth and no alteration in lung function (Yassa, Prosser and Dodge, 1978; Yassa, 1979).

Table VII gives some guidelines on newer dietary supplements for increased calorie and protein intake. Suitable amounts will vary from patient to patient and guidance should be sought from a dietitian. Calculation of total calorie intake is essential: *absorbed* energy intakes of 100—110 per cent are necessary in order to achieve a normal rate of weight gain (Parsons et al, 1983).

Other techniques of supplementary nutrition

More recent attempts have involved *'nasogastric'* and *'nasojejunal'* tube feeding; 'gastrostomy' and 'jejunostomy' tube feeding (the tube is introduced directly into the stomach or jejunum, via the abdominal wall, during a small surgical procedure under general anaesthetic) and *parenteral,* or intravenous, feeding.

Nasogastric and nasojejunal feeding Feeding is usually overnight, using a pump and very fine tubes. Good weight gains have been reported. Shepherd et al (1983) treated seven CF children over six months, using a peptide (protein) formula, giving this either as an oral supplement or as an overnight intragastric tube feed. Total calorie intakes were 120—140 per cent of the recommended daily allowance. With this supplement, significant catch up weight and height gains were observed as well as an increase in body muscle (protein) mass.

Gastrostomy and jejunostomy feeding Although the tubes are commonly left in place for long periods, feeds are usually given at night. Again, gratifying results have been achieved, but longer term evaluation is required.

Parenteral (intravenous) nutrition This is a considerable undertaking. Shepherd, Cooksley and Cooke (1980) observed a catch up in weight and height, after a three week period of feeding, which persisted at six months. Other workers, however, have found more transient improvements (Mansell et al, 1984).

MANAGEMENT OF ASSOCIATED NUTRITIONAL DISORDERS

Lactose intolerance

A small proportion of patients with cystic fibrosis also suffer from lactase deficiency. Management involves omitting lactose from the diet (Antonowicz et al, 1968).

Coeliac disease

An association between cystic fibrosis and coeliac disease has been reported in the literature and observed on other occasions. It is difficult to know whether this is real or apparent (Berg, Dahlqvist and Lindberg, 1979) but coeliac disease should certainly be thought of in young children with cystic fibrosis who fail to thrive on an adequate diet and pancreatic supplements and whose respiratory disease is under control. If coeliac disease is confirmed by jejunal biopsy, a gluten-free diet is indicated.

Diabetes mellitus

In older patients, diabetes mellitus may develop (Chapter 7). It is usually controlled fairly easily and ketoacidosis is not a problem. Management is with diet, oral agents or insulin, along conventional lines.

REFERENCES AND GENERAL READING

Nutrition and dietary management

Antonowicz I, Reddy V, Khaw K-T et al. Lactase deficiency in patients with cystic fibrosis. *Pediatrics 1968; 42:* 492–500

Berg NO, Dahlqvist A, Lindberg T. Exocrine pancreatic insufficiency, small intestinal dysfunction and protein intolerance. A chance occurrence or connection? *Acta Paediatr Scand 1979; 68:* 275–276

Boyer PH. Low birth weight in fibrocystic disease of the pancreas. *Pediatrics 1955; 16:* 778–784

Cox KL, Isenberg JN, Ament ME. Gastric acid hypersecretion in cystic fibrosis. *J Pediatr Gastroenterol Nutr 1982; 1:* 559–565

Crozier DN. Cystic fibrosis. A not-so-fatal disease. *Pediatr Clin North Am 1974; 21:* 943–946

Davidson GP, Hassel FM, Crozier D et al. Iatrogenic hyperuricemia in children with cystic fibrosis. *J Pediatr 1978; 93:* 976–978

Dinwiddie R. The management of the first years of life. In Hodson ME, Norman AP, Batten JC, eds. *Cystic Fibrosis, chapter 11*. London: Bailliere Tindall. 1983: 197–208

Dodge JA. The nutritional state and nutrition. *Acta Paediatr Scand (suppl) 1985:* in press

Durie PR, Bell L, Linton W et al. Effect of cimetidine and sodium bicarbonate on pancreatic replacement therapy in cystic fibrosis. *Gut 1980a; 21:* 778–786

Durie PR, Newth CJ, Forstner et al. Malabsorption of medium chain triglycerides in infants with cystic fibrosis: correction with pancreatic enzyme supplements. *J Pediatr 1980b; 96:* 862–864

Goodchild MC, Sagaro E, Brown GA et al. Comparative trial of Pancrex V forte and Nutrazym in the treatment of malabsorption in cystic fibrosis. *Br Med J 1974; 2:* 712–714

Gow R, Bradbear R, Francis P et al. Comparative study of varying regimens to improve steatorrhoea and creatorrhoea in cystic fibrosis: effectiveness of an enteric-coated preparation with and without antacids and cimetidine. *Lancet 1981; ii:* 1071–1074

Gracey M, Burke V, Anderson CM. Medium chain triglycerides in paediatric practice. *Arch Dis Childh 1970; 45:* 445–452

Harris R, Norman AP, Payne WW. The effect of pancreatic therapy on fat absorption and nitrogen retention in children with fibrocystic disease of the pancreas. *Arch Dis Childh 1955; 30:* 424–427

Kraemer R, Rudeberg A, Hadorn B et al. Relative underweight in cystic fibrosis and its prognostic value. *Acta Paediatr Scand 1978; 67:* 33–37

Laing SC. The nutritional management of children with cystic fibrosis. *J Hum Nutr: Appl Nutr 1985:* in press

Lapey A, Kattwinkel J, di Sant'Agnese PA et al. Steatorrhea and azotorrhea and their relation to growth and nutrition in adolescents and young adults with cystic fibrosis. *J Pediatr 1974; 84:* 328–334

MacDonald A. High, moderate or low fat diets for cystic fibrosis. In *Cystic Fibrosis: Horizons. Proceedings of the 9th International Cystic Fibrosis Congress, Brighton, England.* Chichester: John Wiley and Sons. 1984: 395

Mearns MB. Growth and development. In Hodson ME, Norman AP, Batten JC, eds. *Cystic Fibrosis.* London: Bailliere Tindall. 1983: 183–196

Shepherd RW, Thomas BJ, Bennett D et al. Changes in body composition and muscle protein degradation during nutritional supplementation in nutritionally growth-retarded children with cystic fibrosis. *J Ped Gastroenterol Nutr 1983; 2:* 439–446

Shwachman H. Cystic fibrosis. *Curr Probl Pediatr 1978; VIII (No 10):* 44

Zentler-Munro P. Gastrointestinal disease in adults. In Hodson ME, Norman AP, Batten JC, eds. *Cystic Fibrosis.* London: Bailliere Tindall. 1983: 144–163

Bile acid metabolism

Boyle BJ, Long WB, Balistreri WF et al. Effect of cimetidine and pancreatic enzymes on serum and faecal bile acids and fat absorption in cystic fibrosis. *Gastroenterology 1980; 78:* 950–953

Regan PT, Malageleda JR, Dimagno EP et al. Reduced intraluminal bile acid concentrations and fat maldigestion in pancreatic insufficiency: correction by treatment. *Gastroenterology 1979; 77:* 285–289

Roy CC, Weber AM, Morin CL. Hepatobiliary disease in cystic fibrosis: a survey of current issues and concepts. *J Pediatr Gastroenterol Nutr 1982; 1:* 469–478

Smalley CA, Brown GA, Parkes MET et al. Reduction of bile acid loss in cystic fibrosis by dietary means. *Arch Dis Childh 1978; 53:* 477–482

Watkins JB, Tercyak AM, Szczepanik P et al. Bile salt kinetics in cystic fibrosis: influence of pancreatic enzyme replacement. *Gastroenterology 1977; 73:* 1023–1028

Weber AM, Roy CC, Morin CL et al. Malabsorption of bile acids in children with cystic fibrosis. *N Engl J Med 1973; 289:* 1001–1005

Zentler-Munro PL, Fine DR, Gannon M et al. Effect of cimetidine on intraluminal bile-acid precipitation, pancreatin inactivation and lipid solubilization in pancreatic steatorrhoea. *Gut 1981; 22:* A431

Vitamin supplements

Congden PJ, Bruce G, Rothburn et al. Vitamin status in treated patients with cystic fibrosis. *Arch Dis Childh 1981; 56:* 708–714

Elias E, Muller DPR, Scott J. Association of spinocerebellar disorders with cystic fibrosis or chronic childhood cholestasis and very low serum vitamin E. *Lancet 1981; ii:* 1319–1321

Mineral supplements

Ater JL, Herbst JJ, Landaw SA et al. Relative anaemia and iron deficiency in cystic fibrosis. *Pediatrics 1983; 71:* 810–814

Lloyd-Still JD, Ganther HE. Selenium and glutathione peroxidase levels in cystic fibrosis. *Pediatrics 1980; 65:* 1010–1012

Neve J, van Geffel R, Hanocq M et al. Plasma and erythrocyte zinc, copper and selenium in cystic fibrosis. *Acta Paediatr Scand 1983; 72:* 437–440

van Caillie-Bertrand M de Bieville F, Neijens H et al. Trace metals in cystic fibrosis. *Acta Paediatr Scand 1982; 71:* 203–207

Essential fatty acids

Chase HP, Long MA, Lavin MH. Cystic fibrosis and malnutrition. *J Pediatr 1979; 95:* 337–347

Goodchild MC, Laing S, Custance J et al. Essential fatty acid supplementation: absorption and metabolism. In *Cystic Fibrosis: Horizons. Proceedings of the 9th International CF Congress in Brighton, England.* Chichester: John Wiley and Sons. 1984: 409

Kussoffsky E, Strandvik B, Troell S. Prospective study of fatty acid supplementation over 3 years in patients with cystic fibrosis. *J Pediatr Gastroent Nutr 1983; 2:* 434–438

Rosenlund ML, Lim HK, Kritchevsky K. Essential fatty acids in cystic fibrosis. *Nature 1974; 251:* 719

Nutritional supplementation

Allan JD, Mason A, Moss AD. Nutritional supplementation in treatment of cystic fibrosis of the pancreas. *Am J Dis Child 1973; 126:* 22–26

Lawson D, ed. Gastrointestinal tract, therapy and nutrition. In *Cystic Fibrosis: Horizons. Proceedings of the 9th International CF Congress in Brighton, England.* Chichester: John Wiley and Sons. 1984: 384–391

Mansell AL, Andersen JC, Muttart CR et al. Short-term pulmonary effects of total parenteral nutrition in children with cystic fibrosis. *J Pediatr 1984; 104:* 700–705

Parsons HG, Beaudry P, Dumas A et al. Energy needs and growth in children with cystic fibrosis. *J Pediat Gastroent Nutr 1983; 2:* 44–49

Shepherd RW, Cooksley WGE, Cooke WDD. Improved growth and clinical, nutritional, and respiratory changes in response to nutritional therapy in cystic fibrosis. *J Pediatr 1980; 97:* 351–357

Yassa JG. Growth and nutrition in cystic fibrosis and the effect of an artificial diet. *PhD Thesis, Wales 1979*

Yassa JG, Prosser R, Dodge JA. Effects of an artificial diet on growth of patients with cystic fibrosis. *Arch Dis Childh 1978; 53:* 777–783

Reviews

Bernard O, Alvarez F, Brunelle F et al. Portal hypertension in children. *Clin Gastroenterol 1985; 14:* 33–35

Dodge JA. Nutrition. In Hodson ME, Norman AP, Batten JC, eds. *Cystic Fibrosis.* London: Bailliere Tindall. 1983: 132–143

Francis DEM. Diets for children with cystic fibrosis. In Wrigley M, ed. *Low Fat Diet Cookery Book.* London: Cystic Fibrosis Research Trust. 1983: 59

Hubbard VS, Mangrum PJ. Energy intake and genetic counselling in cystic fibrosis. *J Am Diet Assoc 1982; 80:* 127–131

Park RW, Grand RJ. Gastrointestinal manifestations of cystic fibrosis: a review. *Gastroenterology 1981; 81:* 1143–1161

Chapter 7

MANAGEMENT OF GASTROINTESTINAL AND OTHER COMPLICATING FEATURES

MECONIUM ILEUS

Approximately one in ten of infants affected by CF presents at birth with symptoms of small gut obstruction due to sticky, inspissated intestinal contents. The pathology of this has been described on page 20. The degree of obstruction is very variable: there may be just a delay in the passage of meconium or there may be frank intestinal obstruction *(meconium ileus)*, further complicated, in more than 50 per cent of cases, by volvulus, atresia or perforation with peritonitis.

Clinical features

The typical clinical picture, on the first or second day of life, is one of abdominal distension and bile-stained vomiting. The baby may pass one or two small, white or grey, thick, mucousy bowel motions but usually passes none at all. The diagnosis is simplified if there is already a family history.

Differential diagnosis includes Hirschsprung's disease, small bowel atresia and other rarer causes of obstruction. Most unusually, meconium ileus or an apparently identical disorder occurs in the absence of CF.

Plain X-rays of the abdomen show distended loops of small gut above the obstruction and a mottled appearance, usually in the right lower quadrant, which is due to a mixture of air and inspissated meconium (Figure 22). When this is seen in conjunction with the uneven dilatation of the small gut and there is paucity of fluid levels (because of the sticky nature of the gut contents) the diagnosis of meconium ileus can be made with certainty (Astley, 1986).

If perforation of the bowel has occurred antenatally, flecks of calcified material may be visible on the abdominal film.

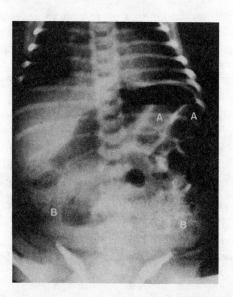

Figure 22. Meconium ileus. Plain X-ray of an infant, showing distended loops of small gut (A,A) and a mottled appearance in the lower quadrants (B,B) which is due to a mixture of air and inspissated meconium

Laboratory tests

None is satisfactory for the diagnosis of CF *at this stage,* with this type of presentation.

Meconium albumin content may be raised in a number of conditions causing neonatal obstruction, apart from CF.

The sweat test is not a particularly good test in the neonatal period (see page 162) although very elevated sodium and chloride levels (more than 90mmol/L) are very suggestive.

Perhaps the most useful and easily obtainable test for supporting the working diagnosis of cystic fibrosis in the newborn is the *serum immunoreactive trypsin (IRT)* but for unknown reasons this may be negative in meconium ileus. Again a *positive* result is suggestive of CF.

Immediate management of CF babies with meconium ileus

If intestinal obstruction is suspected the baby should be transferred immediately from the maternity ward and placed under the joint care of a paediatric surgeon and the paediatrician. It is important to treat not only the obstruction **but all other aspects of CF and this should be instituted without delay.**

Immediate attention should be paid to the infant's hydration. CF babies are very susceptible to the effects of dehydration and electrolyte loss, which lead to thickening of mucus secretions and the development of pulmonary symptoms. Fluid and electrolyte replacement may be needed before any diagnostic or therapeutic measures are undertaken.

Immediate investigations should include: throat swab (cough swab if available), chest X-ray, serum electrolyte levels, sweat test and serum immunoreactive trypsin tests as described above.

Immediate therapy should include: antistaphylococcal antibiotic therapy, vitamin K by injection and chest physiotherapy.

Following careful assessment of the baby and of the abdominal X-ray, *non-operative procedures to expel the meconium* should be considered.

Management of intestinal obstruction

(A) Conservative management

Water-soluble radio-opaque contrast enemas are the method of choice in the uncomplicated case (i.e. in about 50 per cent of the total number of cases) and are successful in about 75 per cent of these. The method used was described first by Noblett (1969). *Gastrografin* is a water soluble iodinated contrast medium. It consists of sodium and methyl glucamine diatrizoates (substances of high osmolality) wetting and flavouring agents. It is introduced per rectum and run up through the colon until it meets the obstruction in the ileum. The colon itself is usually small and empty due to disuse ('microcolon', Figure 23). A forceful expulsion of meconium, gastrografin and fluid usually follows within a few hours and continues over the next 48 hours. The procedure may need to be repeated.

Gastrografin acts by withdrawing fluid from the circulation into the bowel lumen and the meconium mass, and in addition the wetting

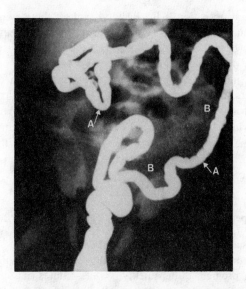

Figure 23. Abdominal X-ray of another CF infant, showing the small colon ('microcolon', arrows A,A) often associated with meconium ileus and outlined by the radio-opaque gastrografin enema. Very distended loops of small gut (B,B), containing meconium, show the characteristic mottled appearance

agent may allow the mass to move along the bowel more freely. The following criteria must be fulfilled:

(a)   no clinical or radiological evidence of surgical complications such as volvulus, atresia or perforation should be present;

(b)   adequate fluid and electrolyte replacement is needed and this should be given by intravenous drip;

(c)   the enema must be fluoroscopically controlled;

(d)   the technique must be done carefully and under close surgical supervision (Noblett, 1969).

It is emphasized that **large amounts of intravenous fluid are necessary and must be carefully monitored** if the baby is to avoid serious dehydration during the procedure.

(B) Operative management

The standard operation is the Bishop-Koop or 'chimney pot' procedure (Bishop and Koop, 1957). The small gut is divided and any gangrenous, atretic or very dilated small gut is excised. The distal portion is thoroughly irrigated, in order to remove as much as possible of the inspissated material; the proximal small gut is then joined to the distal, in an end-to-side fashion, and the distal portion is brought to the surface as an ileostomy. In this way, gut continuity is restored, but opportunity is also provided for washouts to be continued post-operatively. Initially, much of the stool is passed via the ileostomy; later all the stool passes per rectum. At this stage, a second, minor operation is performed and the ileostomy is closed.

(C) Post-operative management

Antibiotics and physiotherapy should be continued.

Many infants who have been treated successfully with gastrografin alone, will progress quite quickly, via clear fluids (nasogastric or oral) to breast milk or cow's milk formulae (see page 100). For those who have had surgery, most will require a period of intravenous parenteral nutrition and will graduate later to one of the modified milks (Pregestimil or Nutramigen) or if possible, to breast-feeding. Lactose-free formulae may be necessary, especially if there has been a significant gut resection.

Pancreatic enzymes are sometimes introduced within a week or two of the first, 'relieving' operation, when ileostomy actions are occurring freely and the baby is tolerating three-hourly feeds. Dosage should be small at first (e.g. Cotazym, half a capsule with alternate feeds). However, some surgeons prefer to wait until the second, 'closing' operation has been done, and excessive numbers of fat globules have been demonstrated in the stools, before starting pancreatic enzymes.

Persistently loose stools may not respond to pancreatin or to lactose-free formulae; loperamide (Imodium), 0.08mg/kg body weight/day may be helpful in these cases.

It is essential to keep the parents fully informed throughout. Separation of mother and infant should be avoided whenever possible by providing accommodation for the mother to stay at the hospital.

Long-term outlook for meconium ileus babies

Meconium ileus complicated by substantial gut resection and other abnormalities has a poorer prognosis than that of CF babies in general, but meconium ileus on its own does not, especially if non-operative techniques can overcome the obstruction. If such babies survive the initial illness (and the vast majority do) their ultimate prognosis is at least as good as that of other CF infants.

'Meconium plug syndrome'

This is not a specific feature of CF. Some infants, particularly the premature, have difficulty in expelling meconium during the first 24 to 48 hours, after which the first stool passed is a colourless or green, thick hard plug, followed by normal meconium. Such babies should have a sweat test to exclude CF and Hirschsprung's disease should also be considered.

MECONIUM ILEUS EQUIVALENT

This is a curious complication in which faecal matter, mixed with stiff, tenacious mucus, collects in masses within the intestinal lumen, most often in the region of the caecum and terminal ileum. It was first described by Jensen (1962).

Clinical features

These include colicky abdominal pain, a palpable mass often in the right lower quadrant of the abdomen which is sometimes tender, and an obstructive element, which if severe, causes abdominal distension, vomiting, constipation and fluid levels on plain abdominal X-ray (see Figure 11, page 39).

Symptoms can occur from about the age of four years and become more common with increasing age. Overall, about 10 per cent of the CF population is affected. Some patients are particularly prone.

The occurrence of meconium ileus equivalent does not relate to the severity of CF in other respects and patients are often in good general health.

Despite its name, meconium ileus equivalent is not necessarily related in cause to meconium ileus of the newborn and nor do these babies show a clearly increased incidence of meconium ileus equivalent in later life.

Precipitating factors are not at all clear, but dehydration, poor control of pancreatic enzyme insufficiency, sudden withdrawal of pancreatic enzymes and dietary indiscretions have all been suggested.

Treatment

Mild episodes, expressed mainly as abdominal pain, will respond to adequate hydration and adjustment of pancreatic enzyme dosage (usually up rather than down).

More severe symptoms will require oral laxatives, e.g. lactulose (Duphalac) or mineral oil (liquid paraffin) and/or simple enemas. In addition, oral mucolytic agents, such as 10 per cent or 20 per cent n-acetyl cysteine (Airbron), 5–10ml four times daily in orange juice, or more palatably, n-acetyl cysteine in granules (Fabrol) (children 1–2 years, one sachet daily; 2–6 years, one sachet twice daily; older children and adults, one sachet 3–4 times daily) taken over weeks or months, may be effective.

Patients with symptoms of obstruction will require admission to hospital, intravenous fluids, intermittent nasogastric suction, simple analgesics and either Airbron or Gastrografin (occasionally both) given orally or by nasogastric tube and by enema. The dosage of n-acetyl cysteine (Airbron) which has been recommended for adults is 30ml of the 20 per cent solution, three times daily, by mouth or nasogastric tube, and 30ml in normal saline by enema, three times daily (Hodson, Mearns and Batten, 1976). The foot of the bed should be placed on high blocks so that the fluid passes along the colon into the caecum. The regime should be continued over several days until bowel evacuation has been as complete as possible and most of the palpable masses have gone.

If Airbron is ineffective, Gastrografin may be tried (Matseshe, Go and DiMagno, 1977; Hanly and Fitzgerald, 1983), preferably under fluoroscopic control and with the same precautions with regard to dehydration (see above). Volumes of Gastrografin which have been suggested are 30ml three times daily orally and 100ml three times daily by enemas, although we have frequently found that much larger doses (for adults) are necessary by mouth or nasogastric tube, and are well tolerated.

Surgery should be avoided if at all possible as this is not only unhelpful in the treatment of meconium ileus equivalent, but may lead to a permanent faecal fistula if the bowel is opened.

Once the acute episode has resolved, oral mucolytic agents should be continued for weeks, months or even longer and attempts should be made to improve the patient's steatorrhoea by giving more effective pancreatic enzyme preparation and dosage (see page 92), possibly with regular cimetidine.

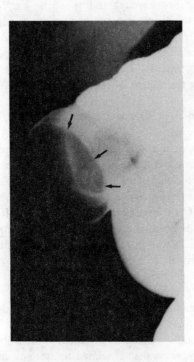

Figure 24. Intussusception — 'spot' film taken during a barium enema. The film shows the abrupt termination of the barium column at the hepatic flexure and 'coiled spring' appearance (arrows) typical of an ileo-colic intussusception. (The 'lead-point' of the intussusception had been located originally at the splenic flexure, and had been reduced by the hydrostatic pressure of the barium suspension, to the hepatic flexure; however complete reduction could not be achieved and surgery was subsequently necessary)

Differential diagnosis of meconium ileus equivalent

Intussusception and **appendicitis/appendix abscess** are the most common. Both may be a complication of meconium ileus equivalent, although this is perhaps more likely in the case of an intussusception, one of the sludge-like masses at the ileo-caecal valve acting as a lead-point. *It can be very difficult to distinguish these conditions, which can all produce pain and a mass in the right iliac fossa.*

Intussusception often provokes quite *severe* intermittent pain, sometimes over several days and the mass may be felt only intermittently. Rectal bleeding may or may not occur. The white blood count is usually normal or only slightly raised. A *diagnostic barium enema* if typical, will show the 'coiled spring' appearance of an intussusception (Figure 24). The radiologist will then attempt a gentle reduction using the weight of the barium, but if this fails, surgery will be required.

Intussusception is a recognized presentation of cystic fibrosis and can occur at any age.

Appendicitis or **appendix abscess** rather than meconium ileus equivalent, are suggested if there is persistently marked local tenderness, fever and a raised white cell count. A policy of nasogastric aspiration and intravenous fluids, over a 12–24 hour period, may help to clarify the situation. If not, operation will be necessary. If appendicitis is not found and the diagnosis is meconium ileus equivalent, a careful attempt should be made to move the masses on manually, but the bowel should not be opened for their removal.

Other conditions which may cause recurrent abdominal pain

Peptic ulcer is said to occur more frequently in CF although the evidence is scanty. If epigastric pain is related to meals it may be worth trying the effect of cimetidine, even before carrying out a barium meal examination.

Recurrent acute pancreatitis is an unusual problem encountered only among those cases of CF who have some residual pancreatic function. Attacks have been provoked by fatty meals and alcohol. Conventional treatment for acute pancreatitis may help, including antacids.

RECTAL PROLAPSE

This is a problem of the preschool child and is uncommon after the age of six years. It occurs in children with bulky stools, even in the absence of a cough, but bouts of coughing may precipitate its appearance. Other contributing factors are poor muscle tone with distension of the large bowel, malnutrition and occasionally, constipation. The prolapse is usually partial, involving the mucosa only.

Rectal prolapse can be a presenting symptom of CF and *its appearance in a young child should be considered as due to CF until a sweat test proves otherwise.*

Management

Immediate treatment consists of lying the child in the head down position and gently encouraging the everted mucosa to reduce with a lubricated gloved finger. Sedation may be needed and reduction may take several hours. **Operative intervention is not necessary.**

Long-term treatment consists of more energetic measures to treat the chest infection (and so the cough) and also to improve the bowel actions, by giving adequate and more effective pancreatin supplements (see page 92). Reduction of total dietary fat, or replacement of some of it with medium chain triglyceride (MCT, page 99) may be useful also. In the rare case of the constipated child, the situation should respond to decreased pancreatin dosage, possibly with use of mineral oil or lactulose.

LIVER DISEASE

Histological evidence of liver damage has been recorded at all ages, from the preterm baby until adult life. These changes, which begin with bile duct plugging and biliary hyperplasia, progress to focal biliary cirrhosis which later becomes multifocal and the liver lobulated, hard and shrunken.

Fatty infiltration also occurs, particularly in those patients who have had prolonged periods of protein/calorie malnutrition.

A more detailed description of pathological changes in the hepatobiliary tract and of abnormalities of bile acid metabolism, is given in Chapter 2, page 18.

From a practical point of view, liver disease sufficiently defined to affect CF patients' well being is found in about 10 per cent of older patients.

The rate of progression of liver change is immensely variable and impossible to predict. In general, progression is slow. It is not known why there is such a variation, nor why cirrhosis develops in the first place. It is not related to the severity of other features of CF and often occurs in patients with good pulmonary status.

Serological liver function tests usually remain within normal limits until considerable liver cirrhosis has occurred (Feigelson, Pecau and Sauvegran, 1970); although some tests are more discriminating than others (Kattwinkel et al, 1973). *Prolongation of prothrombin time* is one of the most sensitive indices of liver disease, but it may also result from malabsorption of vitamin K.

Manifestations of liver disease in CF include prolonged neonatal jaundice, biliary cirrhosis and portal hypertension, liver failure and ascites, hypersplenism and gallstones.

Neonatal cholestasis

Prolonged neonatal jaundice (obstructive in type) is found in few CF babies, except those with meconium ileus, of whom about 50 per cent are affected (Valman, France and Wallis, 1971). The reason for this association is not known. Cholestasis jaundice is an occasional complication of prolonged parenteral nutrition.

Liver biopsy if carried out (this is rarely necessary) shows bile stasis.

Adequate hydration is usually associated with a slow, complete resolution (sometimes over three to four months). If not, a course of oral corticosteroids may be helpful. Abnormalities of prothrombin time should be treated with vitamin K (water soluble if given orally).

Biliary cirrhosis and portal hypertension

This, together with liver failure and ascites, is the most serious outcome of liver disease in CF and affects less than 10 per cent of older patients. **Clinical signs** include hepatosplenomegaly, with eventual regression of the liver. Hypersplenism may occur also, with haematological abnormalities. Presentation is either by clinical signs of hepatic or splenic enlargement, or by bleeding from oesophageal or gastric varices (haematemesis and melaena) or by liver failure and ascites.

Treatment is not very satisfactory. There is no known way of preventing liver damage. When cirrhosis is established, *alcohol* and particularly *aspirin* should be avoided (the latter because of its eroding effect on gastric and oesophageal mucosa, where varices may be present).

Haematemesis from bleeding varices should be treated conservatively at first, with sedation (diazepam is useful), intramuscular vitamin K and transfusion of fresh blood, followed if unsuccessful by intravenous argipressin (Pitressin), 5–20 units in 100ml of 5% dextrose over 15 minutes or 0.4 units/minute for a maximum of two hours. In most instances, bleeding will cease with this regime. Cimetidine should be given in the recovery period.

On rare occasions, a Senstaken-Blakemore tube may be necessary, as a temporary measure.

When bleeding has settled, consideration should be given to *obliteration of the varices by injection of a sclerosing agent,* under direct vision via a flexible endoscope. The injections are repeated at two to six week intervals until all the large vessels are sclerosed (Psacharopoulos et al, 1981). This technique has been associated with less morbidity than other, more complicated surgical procedures (Stamatakis et al, 1982) and follow-up has been regarded as satisfactory over four years so far (Psacharopoulos and Mowat, 1983).

Massive bleeding may require emergency surgical treatment by ligation of varices, with oesophageal or gastric transection and stapling. However, even in these circumstances, repeated sclerotherapy and the use of a Senstaken tube may be effective (Psacharopoulos and Mowat, 1983).

Portosystemic shunting operations have been carried out, to relieve the pressure within the liver (Schuster et al, 1977) but these are formidable procedures and results overall have not been very impressive.

In deciding whether heroic measures such as oesophageal/gastric transection and stapling, or shunt operations are indicated, the patient's probable long-term survival should be taken into account, with reference to his respiratory condition.

Liver failure and ascites

This alternative presentation will require treatment with a low protein intake, *some* sodium restriction, oral neomycin or lactulose to decrease the nitrogen and ammonia production within the gut, and the cautious use of a potassium-sparing diuretic, such as spironolactone (Aldactone) starting at low dosage. Chlorothiazide (Saluric) again in low dosage, may be added if necessary. (Paradoxically, sodium chloride supplements (e.g. slow sodium, Ciba) may be necessary if spironolactone induces a state of sodium depletion.)

Hypersplenism

The rare complication of massive splenic enlargement, with haemato-logical abnormalities and infarction, occasionally occurs and can cause dragging abdominal pain.

Gallstones

These may be symptomatic in older patients and require removal. Shwachman and Grand (1978) found that they were present in as many as 12 per cent of patients overall, but they were only symptomatic in about two per cent.

Although liver disease with its ramifications is unremitting and difficult to treat its recognition need not cause too much despondency: in many patients, the progression is very slow, over several years, during which most of those afflicted continue to live virtually normal lives.

DIABETES MELLITUS

There is a well recognized disorder which is probably a complication (rather than an association) of CF. It appears in overt form **in 5–10 per cent of older patients** (an incidence of approximately 5–10 times greater than a population of comparable age) and in sub-clinical form (i.e. an abnormal glucose tolerance test and reduced insulin response to an oral or intravenous glucose load) in 30–50 per cent of patients of all ages.

The aetiology of the diabetes is not well established but pancreatic fibrosis with gradual impairment of blood supply to the islets of Langer-hans is a possible explanation. The impaired insulin response is improved with a sulphonylurea (glibenclamide) indicating that at least part of the explanation is a defective insulin release from the islet cells. It is debat-able whether there is any abnormality of glucagon release in CF subjects

(Redmond, Buchanan and Trimble, 1977; Lippe, Sperling and Dooley, 1977).

The diabetes of CF is usually controlled without much difficulty and ketoacidosis is rare. Late complications such as retinopathy, neuropathy and renal disease are not unknown but the incidence appears to be very low.

The diagnosis of diabetes should always be considered if a patient has an unexplained weight loss. A history may reveal other relevant symptoms, such as polyuria, polydypsia and an altered appetite. **Urine testing for glucose should be carried out at regular intervals in older patients.**

Management

Most patients will require insulin but for some younger ones, oral hypoglycaemic agents are sufficient. Measurement of glycosylated haemoglobin values (Hb 1Ac) may be useful in achieving better control.

The help of a dietitian should be sought to reconcile the management of diabetes with the increased nutritional requirements of cystic fibrosis.

DELAYED PUBERTY

A delay of about two years, on average, is to be expected except in those with minimal lung disease. However, normal sexual development occurs eventually, in both sexes and maturation is complete by late teenage, even in those with very delayed puberty (Holsclaw et al, 1971; Moshang and Holsclaw, 1980; Reiter, Stern and Root, 1981).

Bone age is also delayed and correlates with stature and sexual development. It is helpful to point out to worried adolescents that they *will* mature and that their growth will continue when their peers have reached adult height.

FERTILITY

Involvement of the vas deferens (page 23) means that **the majority of affected males are infertile**, although sexual potency is not impaired. However fertility in CF males has been reported (Feigelson, Pecau and Shwachman, 1969; Taussig et al, 1972; Blanck and Mendoza, 1976) and a sperm count should be done before sterility is assumed. Young men often become distressed when they discover that they are unlikely to produce children of their own and need careful and sympathetic counselling. It must be emphasized that *fertility although unlikely, is possible* and that sexual activity is not affected.

In the female, fertility may be *slightly* impaired, the thick cervical mucus possibly presenting an impediment to the passage of spermatozoa (Oppenheimer and Esterly, 1970). A survey in the USA and Canada (Cohen, di Sant'Agnese and Friedlander, 1980) among 100 CF women, revealed that 97 of 129 pregnancies were 'completed' (that is, they were not lost by miscarriage, either spontaneous or therapeutic) and that 86 viable infants were born, of whom only one had CF. There was an increased incidence of preterm infants. The one CF baby among the 85 normal ones (there were no other congenital abnormalities) was in keeping with the empirical risk of a CF mother having an affected child, that is 1 : 40–1 : 50.

Pregnancy in CF women

This has not been recommended for those with Shwachman scores below 80 (see page 151) as considerable deterioration of pulmonary disease may occur (Cohen et al, 1980). Nevertheless, this same survey of CF women, which included many patients with lower scores, showed that maternal mortality rate did not exceed those expected for CF women of the same age.

Pregnancy in CF women requires particularly careful antenatal management with meticulous attention to the various complicating factors. This care should be undertaken jointly by the obstetrician and the patient's usual specialist physician.

Breast-feeding has been accomplished successfully by at least one CF mother (Welch, Phelps and Osher, 1981) and the salt content of this milk was normal. Reports of salt content in CF breast milk have varied and the milk should be analysed if breast-feeding is contemplated.

Contraception

The near-normal fertility of CF women creates a need for effective contraception. In most cases, this is best supplied by the oral contraceptive oestrogen/progesterone 'pill' although dosage may have to be greater than usual to take into account the effects of malabsorption and anti-biotics. Blood progesterone levels should be checked on day 21 after starting the 'pill' to establish whether hormone dosage derived from the 'pill' has been sufficiently high to suppress ovulation.

A 'barrier' method of protection, although less reliable, may be more appropriate for a few patients who have established liver disease.

JOINT PROBLEMS

During the last 20 years or so, a number of different joint problems have been recognized in CF, apparently associated in some way with the disease.

Hypertrophic pulmonary osteoarthropathy (HPOA) has been mentioned in Chapter 5, page 77. Clinically the condition affects large

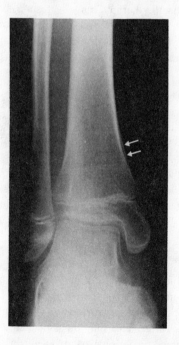

Figure 25. Hypertrophic pulmonary osteoarthropathy (HPOA) in a CF patient aged 17 years. This X-ray, showing the lower ends of the tibia and fibula with the ankle, illustrates the periosteal new bone formation (arrows)

joints, e.g. ankles and knees, sometimes with an effusion (Grossman, Denning and Baker, 1964; Braude et al, 1984). Radiologically, there is periostitis and new bone formation (Figure 25).

A more acute form of transient synovitis has been reported in younger patients (Newman and Ansell, 1979).

All varieties settle with symptomatic treatment, e.g. with ibuprofen (Brufen) or paracetamol. Aspirin is not recommended in CF, especially in older patients, because of the possibility of co-existent liver disease with varices (see page 118).

SALT DEPLETION

This is rarely a problem in the United Kingdom with its temperate climate, although precipitating factors such as gastroenteritis, or any febrile illness can produce an increased requirement for salt. Occasionally, prolonged diuretic therapy may be responsible (see page 120). Supplements, when required, are best given at intervals throughout the day, as table salt in feeds or fruit drinks for infants and young children, and as enteric-coated tablets (slow sodium) for older patients.

Dosage

This is approximately: 500mg/day   — up to one year
                        1g/day   — up to seven years
                        2—4g/day   thereafter

Fluids should be taken liberally.

Care should be exercised when cor pulmonale is present, when additional salt may attract an increased circulating fluid load.

CARE OF THE TEETH

Regular toothbrushing, using a fluoride toothpaste and regular visits to the dentist, are as important for the CF patient as for everyone. However, there is a strong clinical impression that CF people show a *decreased incidence of dental caries.* This may be associated with a more alkaline saliva with an increased buffering capacity (Kinirons, 1983).

Staining of teeth due to tetracyclines

The tetracycline group of drugs is well known for their permanent staining effect on the teeth. This can occur following even short courses of treatment given before the age of 12 years.

Cosmetic veneers of tooth-coloured material provide a very adequate temporary solution to the problem, and improve morale. They are appropriate until dentition has matured sufficiently to allow the affected teeth to be crowned, using porcelain jacket crown preparations.

REFERENCES AND GENERAL READING

Meconium ileus

Astley R. In Anderson CM, Burke V, Gracey M, eds. *Paediatric Gastroenterology, 2nd Edition.* Oxford: Blackwell Scientific Publications. In preparation
Bishop HC, Koop CE. Management of meconium ileus: resection, Roux-en-y anastomosis and ileostomy irrigation with pancreatic enzymes. *Ann Surg 1957; 145:* 410–414
Noblett HR. Treatment of uncomplicated meconium ileus by gastrografin enema: a preliminary report. *J Pediat Surg 1969; 4:* 190–197
Wagget J, Johnson DG, Borns P et al. The non-operative treatment of meconium ileus by gastrografin enema. *J Pediat 1970; 77:* 407–411

Meconium ileus equivalent and intussusception

Gracey M, Burke V, Anderson CM. Treatment of abdominal pain in cystic fibrosis by oral administration of n-acetyl cysteine. *Arch Dis Childh 1969; 44:* 404–405
Hanley JG, Fitzgerald MX. Meconium ileus equivalent in older patients with cystic fibrosis. *Br Med J 1983; 1:* 1411–1413
Hodson ME, Mearns MB, Batten JC. Meconium ileus equivalent in adults with cystic fibrosis of pancreas: a report of six cases. *Br Med J 1976; 2:* 790–791
Holsclaw DS, Rocmans C, Shwachman H. Intussusception in patients with cystic fibrosis. *Pediatrics 1971; 48:* 51–58
Jensen KG. Meconium ileus equivalent in a 15-year-old patient with mucoviscidosis. *Acta Paediatr Scand 1962; 51:* 344–348
Matseshe JW, Go VLW, Dimagno EP. Meconium ileus equivalent complicating cystic fibrosis in postneonatal children and young adults. Report of 12 cases. *Gastroenterology 1977; 72:* 732–736
Rosenstein BJ, Langbaum TS. Incidence of distal intestinal obstruction syndrome in cystic fibrosis. *J Pediatr Gastroenterol Nutr 1983; 2:* 299–301

Rectal prolapse

Stern RC, Izant RJ, Boat TF et al. Treatment and prognosis of rectal prolapse in cystic fibrosis. *Gastroenterology 1982; 82:* 707–710

Liver disease

Feigelson J, Pecau Y, Cathelineau L et al. Additional data on hepatic function tests in cystic fibrosis. *Acta Paediat Scand 1975; 64:* 337–344

Feigelson J, Pecau Y, Sauvegrain J. Liver function studies and biliary tract investigations in mucoviscidosis. *Acta Paediat Scand 1970; 59:* 539–544

Goodchild MC, Banks AJ, Drolc Z et al. Liver scans in cystic fibrosis. *Arch Dis Childh 1975; 50:* 813–815

Kattwinkel J, Taussig LM, Statland BE et al. The effects of age on alkaline phosphatase and other serological liver function tests in normal subjects and patients with cystic fibrosis. *J Pediatr 1973; 82:* 234–242

Psacharopoulos HT, Howard ER, Portmann B et al. Hepatic complications of cystic fibrosis. *Lancet 1981; ii:* 78–80

Psacharopoulos HT, Mowat AP. The liver and biliary system. In Hodson ME, Norman AP, Batten JC, eds. *Cystic Fibrosis.* London: Bailliere Tindall. 1983: 164–182

Schuster SR, Shwachman H, Toyama WM et al. The management of portal hypertension in cystic fibrosis. *J Ped Surg 1977; 12:* 201–206

Stamatakis JD, Howard ER, Psacharopoulos HT et al. Injection sclerotherapy for oesophageal varices in children. *Br J Surg 1982; 69:* 74–75

Starkey BJ, Goodchild MC. Postprandial total serum bile acid concentrations in cystic fibrosis. *Monogr Paediatr 1979; 10:* 12–18

Valman HB, France NE, Wallis PG. Prolonged neonatal jaundice in cystic fibrosis. *Arch Dis Childh 1971; 46:* 805–809

Diabetes mellitus

Handwerger S, Roth J, Gorden P et al. Glucose intolerance in cystic fibrosis. *N Engl J Med 1969; 281:* 451–461

Lippe BM, Sperling MA, Dooley RR. Pancreatic alpha and beta cell function in cystic fibrosis. *J Pediatr 1977; 90:* 751–755

Milner AD. Blood glucose and serum insulin levels in children with cystic fibrosis. *Arch Dis Childh 1969; 44:* 351–355

Redmond AO, Buchanan KD, Trimble ER. Insulin and glucagon response to arginine infusion in cystic fibrosis. *Acta Paediatr Scand 1977; 16:* 199–204

Rodman HM, Matthews LW. Hyperglycaemia in cystic fibrosis: a review of the literature and own patient experience. In Warwick WJ, ed. *1000 Years of Cystic Fibrosis.* University of Minnesota. 1981: 67–76

Wilmshurst EG, Soeldner JS, Holsclaw DS et al. Endogenous and exogenous insulin responses in patients with cystic fibrosis. *Pediatrics 1975; 55:* 75–82

Fertility and reproduction

Blanck RR, Mendoza EM. Fertility in a man with cystic fibrosis. *JAMA 1976; 235:* 1364

Cohen LF, di Sant'Agnese PA, Friedlander J. Cystic fibrosis and pregnancy. A national survey. *Lancet 1980; ii:* 842–844

Feigelson J, Pecau Y, Shwachman H. Paternity in a patient with mucoviscidosis. Study of genital function and filiation. *Arch Franc Pediatr 1969; 26:* 936–944 (Fr.)

Grand RJ, Talamo RC, di Sant'Agnese PA, Shwartz RH. Pregnancy in cystic fibrosis of the pancreas. *JAMA 1966; 195:* 993–1000

Holsclaw DS, Perlmutter AD, Jockin H et al. Genital abnormalities in male patients with cystic fibrosis. *J Urol 1971; 106:* 568–574

Moshang T, Holsclaw DS. Menarchal determinants in cystic fibrosis. *Am J Dis Child 1980; 134:* 1139–1142

Oppenheimer EH, Esterly JR. Observation on cystic fibrosis of the pancreas. VI The uterine cervix. *J Pediatr 1970; 77:* 991–995

Reiter EO, Stern RC, Root AW. The reproductive endocrine system in cystic fibrosis. I Basal gonadotrophin and sex steroid levels. *Am J Dis Child 1981; 135:* 422–426

Taussig LM, Lobeck CC, di Sant'Agnese PA et al. Fertility in males with cystic fibrosis. *N Engl J Med 1972; 287:* 586–589

Welch MJ, Phelps DL, Osher AB. Breast-feeding by a mother with cystic fibrosis. *Pediatrics 1981; 67:* 664–666

Joint problems

Braude S, Kennedy A, Hodson M et al. Hypertrophic osteoarthropathy in cystic fibrosis. *Br Med J 1984; 288:* 822–823

Grossman H, Denning CR, Baker DH. Hypertrophic osteoarthropathy in cystic fibrosis. *Am J Dis Child 1964; 107:* 1–6

Newman AJ, Ansell BM. Episodic arthritis in children with cystic fibrosis. *J Pediatr 1979; 94:* 594–596

Schidlow DV, Goldsmith DP, Palmer J et al. Arthritis in cystic fibrosis. *Arch Dis Childh 1984; 59:* 377–379

Miscellaneous problems

Aterman K. Duodenal ulceration and fibrocystic pancreas disease. *Am J Dis Child 1961; 101:* 210–215

Hen J, Dolan TF, Touloukian RJ. Meconium plug syndrome associated with cystic fibrosis and Hirschsprung's disease. *Pediatrics 1980; 66:* 466–468

Kinirons MJ. Increased salivary buffering in association with a low caries experience in children suffering from cystic fibrosis. *J Dent Res 1983; 62:* 815–817

Primosch RE. Tetracycline discoloration, enamel defects and dental caries in patients with cystic fibrosis. *Oral Surg 1980; 50:* 301–308

Shwachman H, Lebenthal E, Khaw KT. Recurrent acute pancreatitis in patients with cystic fibrosis with normal pancreatic enzymes. *Pediatrics 1975; 55:* 86–95

Wood RE, Herman CJ, Johnson KW et al. Pneumatosis coli in cystic fibrosis. *Am J Dis Child 1975; 129:* 246–248

Reviews

di Sant'Agnese PA, Davis PB. Cystic fibrosis in adults. 75 cases and a review of 232 cases in the literature. *Am J Med 1979; 66:* 121–129

Mitchell-Heggs P, Mearns MB, Batten JC. Cystic fibrosis in adolescents and adults. *Q J Med 1976; 45:* 479–504

Shwachman H, Grand RJ. Cystic fibrosis. In Sleisenger MH, Fordtran JS, eds. *Gastrointestinal Disease.* Philadelphia: W B Saunders. 1978: 1468

Chapter 8

MANAGEMENT OF THE PATIENT IN THE FAMILY

The improving prognosis of CF has been achieved at considerable cost, both emotionally and financially to the patient and his family, and financially to the medical services. In recent years the social problems of the condition have become almost as important as the medical ones.

'Successful' management' requires an understanding of the disease process and the reason for the many aspects of care by all those involved: doctors, ancillary medical workers, parents and the patient himself, who as he grows up, will wish to manage certain aspects of his own condition. **Consequently, education plays a major role in management.**

MANAGEMENT OF THE NEWLY DIAGNOSED CHILD

The initial handling of the situation when a serious and potentially lethal condition is first diagnosed is extremely difficult and very important. Despite growing interest in CF among the medical profession and scientists in general, the parents of a newly diagnosed child have often never heard of CF or if they have, know little of the implications of the diagnosis.

The first interview

It is perhaps trite to say that the disclosure of any abnormality of more than minor degree is a severe shock to parents and that the manner in which it is done is remembered for the rest of their days. It is certainly so for the parents of the CF child and **their capacity for absorbing information at the first interview is very limited.**

Having established the diagnosis beyond reasonable doubt, arrangements should be made to see **both parents together.**

This arrangement in itself (carried out as soon as practicable after the request has been made) will usually indicate that the matter to be discussed is an important one.

The interview should be conducted by a senior doctor with experience of CF who will be involved in the child's continuing care. It is unfair (to the parents and to the doctor) to delegate such an interview to a junior member of the medical staff, who may try to impart too much knowledge, little of which is assimilated and who may answer difficult questions such as, "how long will he live?" in too definitive a way.

It is necessary to offer the parents other opportunities to discuss the problem. **At the initial interview** although one should be willing to answer particular queries about the child's immediate condition, it is **often sufficient to indicate, in general terms, that CF is a serious disease but one with an improving outlook** as a result of earlier diagnosis and modern treatment.

We think it is best to indicate at this stage that it is inherited, to give some preliminary explanation of this and to explain that it is **inherited equally from both parents.**

Many parents will go away from the first interview to seek knowledge of the disease from books, encyclopaedias and from other people — therefore we find it better to offer an explanatory booklet straight away so that we know that the information they receive will be accurate, up-to-date and not over-dramatized. (The booklet entitled 'Cystic Fibrosis' written by Dr David Lawson for the Cystic Fibrosis Research Trust in the United Kingdom is very useful for this purpose).

Subsequent interviews

Arrangements should be made to see the parents again after a few days when more specific questions may be discussed.

Throughout these interviews **it is appropriate to adopt a hopeful attitude.** However, the seriousness of the disease must be communicated in order to achieve meaningful genetic counselling and co-operation in long-term management. It is also appropriate at this early stage, to mention the following:

1. **CF children are of normal intelligence** and often have a great deal of drive and determination which should always be encouraged;

2. most children go to normal schools;

3. within their limitations, they should take part in normal physical activities;

4. they are not more *susceptible* to infections;

5. they are not infectious;

6. as babies they should be clothed and taken outdoors just as normal babies;

7. they are not going to have different diets from the rest of the family apart from some relatively minor adjustments;

8. they should experience the normal disciplines and standards set by the family as a whole.

From the onset it is important that parents should not overprotect their child; they should try to achieve as normal a life for him as possible within the constraints of medical treatment.

Parents should be asked if they would like to be put in touch with the **Cystic Fibrosis Research Trust** (in the UK) or an equivalent organization in other countries, so that they can receive literature on treatment and research and perhaps make contact with local parents of affected children whose support and advice is often invaluable.

Difficulties occur most frequently in families where:

1. *a fatal prognosis* with mention of a definite age of death, has been given at the initial interview (unfortunately this still seems to be done);

2. *the father is not involved* in explanations and discussions with the mother and doctor from the beginning;

3. *an over-protective attitude* has been allowed to develop from the onset. This is damaging not only for the patient but for the other children in the family.

Discussion of the diagnosis in CF children who are recognized by *screening procedures* (i.e. as young babies, before the onset of significant symptoms, see page 170) presents a somewhat different problem. In such interviews it could be even more important to keep a correct balance between a positive, hopeful approach and an understanding of the seriousness of the diagnosis.

Instruction of parents in treatment procedures

As there are many facets of treatment, including many drugs and physical treatments, it is helpful if parents can participate fully from the beginning. If the patient is in hospital, *it is sensible to ask the mother to stay in hospital with the baby for at least a short period, but preferably throughout,* so that she can learn treatment regimes from members of the health care team — doctors, nurses, physiotherapists, dietitian, and not lose contact with her baby. This also helps her to accept the situation. She should learn the proper names of drugs, understand physiotherapy and inhalation techniques and details of diet etc. The opportunity provided for a more leisurely discussion of the disease can do much to restore confidence in a bewildering situation. *Both parents should be instructed whenever possible.*

GENETIC COUNSELLING

The genetic basis of the disease and the inheritance risks have been described in the first chapter (page 6).

Formal referral to a geneticist is not usually necessary, as CF has a straightforward inheritance pattern (Mendelian recessive). The genetic aspects will be familiar to the child's own paediatrician and his involvement with the family makes him the most appropriate person to discuss the genetics and to advise when invited.

Family understanding of the mode of inheritance

A review of 100 CF families in Scotland and Northern Ireland revealed a poor understanding by the parents of the mode of inheritance and this contributed substantially to the unhappiness; inadequate and badly timed instruction by the diagnosing physician was thought to have been largely responsible (McCrae et al, 1973; Burton, 1975). A similar study of 52 families in Sweden showed that 29 couples were either given incorrect information on inheritance, no information or information which came too late for the parents to prevent another pregnancy (Falkman, 1977).

Even trained geneticists, when reviewing the results of their own counselling to parents, regarding a variety of inherited diseases, find that the majority of parents have a poor understanding of what was discussed with them initially (Harper, 1984).

It does not seem an easy matter to give genetic advice. An assessment must be made of the parents' capacity to understand. On this will depend the degree of scientific detail with which the genetic risks and statistics are given.

Explanations should be made clearly and simply and with the aid of diagrams, preferably drawn during the explanation (see Figure 2, page 7).

When discussing the 1:4 recurrence in sibs it must be stressed that this figure is *theoretical*. Because one, or even two children in a family have CF, it does not follow that the next one will be normal — 'chance has no memory'. For parents who have produced one CF child, *all* further pregnancies carry the 1:4 risk. With the application of recent techniques for antenatal diagnosis (Brock, Bedgood, Barron et al, 1985) it is possible to reduce these risks very considerably — about 90 per cent of CF cases, conceived by known carriers, can now be detected antenatally, with a false positive rate of five per cent. In other words, even with antenatal diagnosis, at the present time, there is still a 10 per cent chance that a pregnant mother is carrying a CF fetus if the result is negative and a smaller risk (5%) that she may agree to the abortion of a normal fetus if the result is positive.

Guilt feelings

One of the prime objects of genetic counselling is to allay any feelings of guilt and shame. Parents often have feelings of guilt which need to be acknowledged and understood. They need reassurance that these are unfounded. The following should always be stressed:

1. everyone in the community carries some recessive genes, one person in 20 carries the CF gene;

2. the inheritance comes equally from both parents;

3. the condition is not related to any antenatal treatment or illness;

4. it bears no proven relationship to other illnesses in parents and grandparents;

5. it is not necessary for there to have been any recognized cases in previous generations.

In summary, nothing the parents could have done before or during the pregnancy could have influenced the development of CF in this child. For the first CF baby of the marriage, for whom antenatal diagnosis is

not available at the moment, CF is unpredictable and unpreventable.
When CF carriers can be identified, this situation will change.

The 'normal children'

The statistical risk that other children in the family are carriers is 2:3,
as set out in Figure 2, page 7. Carriers cannot bear CF children unless
they have the misfortune to marry other carriers and this risk is *their*
risk (2:3) multiplied by the carrier rate in the community (1:20) —
i.e. 1:30. With CF predicted for 1:4 for each of the children of such
marriages, the overall risk that a CF sibling (of unknown carrier status)
will have a CF child is 1:120 or less than one per cent. This figure
compares favourably with the likelihood of any person of unknown
genetic status, having a child with a major abnormality. Healthy CF
siblings should be reassured in answer to their questions on marriage
and the advisability of having children.

Discussion with parents about future pregnancies

Parents' views about future pregnancies are likely to be influenced by
their experience of their first CF child and it is important to emphasise
the great variability in severity of the disease, even within the same
family. They would be wise to postpone pregnancy for at least a year
or two, during which they will have the opportunity to learn more about
the disease and perhaps meet other parents or other CF children before
making up their minds. Their ultimate decision will be their own, but
should be taken in the light of full and frank discussion with their
medical advisors and with assurance of appropriate support whatever
the outcome.

Antenatal diagnosis, available now for known carriers of CF, i.e.
for parents of a CF child, will form an important part of these discussions (see page 8).

Adoption should be discussed. Unfortunately, few children are
offered for adoption these days. It is often more difficult for a family
with a CF child to be able to adopt. Families should discuss their own
particular circumstances with their local authority.

Contraception is probably a better choice than sterilization, especially
for young parents, as future research should improve methods of antenatal diagnosis and eventually, should define the basic defect. In the

meantime fatal accidents and separations do happen. *Adequate family planning advice* should be offered and arranged if necessary.

The occasional family will consider artificial insemination, in the knowledge that there is as yet, no reliable method of heterozygote detection.

If sterilization is chosen, this is available under the National Health Service in the United Kingdom.

SOCIAL AND PSYCHOLOGICAL FACTORS AFFECTING THE PATIENT AND HIS FAMILY

The patient

Several reports have highlighted the psychological problems associated with CF, which can be especially marked in the adolescent (Boyle et al, 1976; Falkman, 1977; Drotar et al, 1981; Bywater, 1981; Sinnema et al, 1983). **These problems are largely related to the effects of chronic ill health** i.e.:

chronic cough with sputum production;
offensive stools with flatulence;
recurrent abdominal pain;
small stature;
delayed appearance of secondary sexual characteristics;
missed schooling;
difficulty in obtaining, and keeping, employment;
reduced marriage prospects;
eventual knowledge of a high likelihood of sterility in the male;
the health danger to the female of having children;
the ultimately fatal nature of the disease.

Many worries are not fully expressed by the patient. They should all be discussed at an appropriate stage. A paediatrician caring for children until they are fully adolescent or adult, should be prepared to train himself to talk to older patients.

A *psychiatrist* may be useful and necessary in certain circumstances particularly for the older patient. It is perhaps surprising how emotionally robust most CF children are (or appear to be) and how well they adjust to their problems (Drotar et al, 1981; Lewis and Khaw, 1982). The older patient, however, may wish to discuss his worries with someone different from the doctor who has known him from babyhood and who has developed a close association with his parents.

A *social worker* can also offer emotional support to patients and families. She can play an important role with the doctor in the discussion of education, employment and relationships with the opposite sex and can advise on appropriate social benefits (see below).

The following factors help to reduce the problems of the adolescent:

1. involvement of the father in the patient's treatment;

2. some outside interests for the mother, compatible with looking after her family;

3. encouragement for the parents to allow greater independence for their son or daughter;

4. opportunity for frank discussion of the patient's problems, both within the home and perhaps with peer groups (Boyle et al, 1976).

Participation in holidays or camps for young people with CF has been beneficial as a means of developing independence and helping the patient to realize that his problems are not unique.

Discussion groups for affected adolescents and adults, conducted by a trusted adult such as a social worker may have a similar good effect (Strauss, Pedersen and Dudovitz, 1979).

Most recently and impressively, CF adults have now formed their own Association and the *First International Cystic Fibrosis (Muscoviscidosis) Young Adults Meeting* took place in Brussels in 1982. Fifteen countries were represented by 40 participants, many of whom presented papers on various aspects of 'living with CF'. These meetings are now held yearly. The Association of CF Adults (UK) publishes a regular newsletter (obtainable on request from the Editors, 288 New Road, Ferndown, Dorset BH22 8EP).

The extended family

The impact of a diagnosis of CF upon other family members can be considerable. Like most serious disorders the condition is associated with an increased incidence of family emotional problems and with family disruption. A marriage which was already unstable may break down more quickly than it might have done. On the other hand, a marriage which was secure before the advent of the CF child is often strengthened by the sharing of the burden; for this if for no other reason the father's full participation in the child's care is very important (Burton, 1975; Falkman, 1977).

The exigencies of treatment and the financial and social complications demand large resources of energy, devotion and good sense. Mothers in particular, can become extremely tired and sometimes depressed (Bywater, 1981; 1984) which can be irksome to the husband and the other children. A fairer distribution of the load among all family members is to everyone's advantage.

It is often hard for parents to balance the time, attention and affection given to *all* their children, and it is good practice for the doctor to enquire about the health and behaviour of siblings and to offer advice if necessary.

EDUCATION

Every effort should be made to provide the CF child with a good education, because this in itself can produce enjoyment and because it has practical value in later years when he is seeking employment.

CF children with well controlled lung disease have little difficulty in meeting the educational and recreational programmes of ordinary schools, but those with more severe lung involvement suffer gradually increasing symptoms and a few need special educational provision. **There is no place however for special education or treatment simply on account of the diagnosis.**

CF children attending normal schools should take part in those physical activities of which they feel capable. Allowances may be necessary during times of ill health.

It is helpful for the parents to discuss the child's condition with the teacher, *preferably before the child enters school* and to offer some CF literature if the teacher is not familiar with the disease.

CF children possess a great deal of drive and initiative. They are not children who sit about doing nothing. Many mothers state that their CF child has more energy than their other children. Often, after missed periods at school, they make up work very quickly. (Naturally, this is not always the case and extra tuition may be required on occasions).

Most CF children will benefit from 'school trips', whether in their own country or abroad. Many adolescents and young adults have travelled the world and taken university courses overseas. Although their ultimate longevity may be shortened by such ventures, mere prolonging of life should not be a reason for limiting these activities.

Home teaching

This can be arranged on a short-term basis to allow the child to catch up with missed schooling and to restore morale, and on a long-term basis for the more seriously and chronically sick. In Great Britain at the present time, the quota of home teaching normally varies between three and eight hours per week with additional work provided for the child to do on his own. An assessment is made of the needs of the individual child. Arrangements vary from county to county.

Employment and career prospects

A suitable choice of employment and career is particularly important for the CF patient, who is generally less fit than other people and more reliant on their goodwill. The matter should be discussed with the child and parents early in teenage.

In both normal and special schools, officers of the National Careers Service offer advice and guidance to all pupils from the age of 14 years. A Specialist Careers Officer is responsible for identifying and assisting handicapped pupils in normal schools. The aim of these services is to place the young person in suitable employment, or if this is not possible immediately, or if he wishes to follow a career, to arrange for a course of instruction, full-time or part-time, which will lead to suitable employment. Grants are available for certain training courses and higher education.

CF patients who have left school, and who have difficulty in obtaining employment, can be helped by the disablement resettlement services. It is sometimes helpful if they register as disabled, although many CF people, understandably, are reluctant to do this. If the procedure can be seen as a means to an end and not as an acknowledgment of disability, it may be accepted.

With regard to choices of employment and careers, a wide variety is open to CF people provided that the work can be done in a reasonably sheltered environment and away from dust and fumes. Some gain places at Universities and Training Colleges. Most cope admirably with many pressures, but is is important that they have rooms of their own, adequately heated, in which to continue physiotherapy and that there is a liaison between the college doctor and the patient's specialist physician.

It is usually desirable for employers to be aware of the diagnosis from the onset and many have an understanding attitude to the necessary absences and hospital admissions. However, regrettably, this is not always the case.

TRANSFER OF MEDICAL CARE FROM
PAEDIATRICIAN TO ADULT PHYSICIAN

This is an area where there is considerable room for improvement.

It is only relatively recently that it has become at all common for such a transfer to be made. Now, sizeable clinics of adult CF patients are being built up and there is an increased awareness of the disease among adult physicians. Owing to the predominant role of chest disease in CF, the adult chest physician is the most appropriate person to take on this subsequent care.

Prolonged survival into late teens and beyond increases the incidence of many of the complications of cystic fibrosis including the psychological ones.

Patients are usually transferred in their late teens and many take badly to the change. By this time, the patient usually understands his disease very fully, as do his parents; a relationship has been built up with the paediatrician over many years, based on trust and experience, which all are reluctant to relinquish. At this time too, patients are keenly aware of the realities of the disease and its ultimately fatal nature. The resultant depression often leads to rejection of treatment. Sometimes there is an element of rejection of their parents also — common enough in adolescents without CF.

It is probably best for the transfer to take place *slowly*. The older paediatric patient should get to know the adult physician during the last year or so before the transfer, by making a series of outpatient visits to him. Even after the transfer has occurred, paediatric and adult physicians should continue to work closely together as a team, if possible holding some joint clinics and sharing ancillary staff. In some countries, there is no sharp distinction between paediatric and adult CF specialists and the same team is able to look after patients at all ages. This has obvious advantages for both patients and health care teams.

Psychological adjustment to cystic fibrosis, particularly at this changeover period, profoundly affects the clinical progress of the patient as outlined in Figure 26.

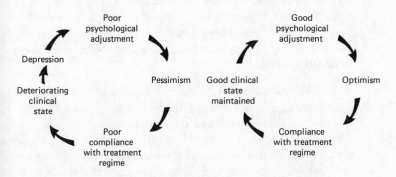

Figure 26. Psychological factors in cystic fibrosis

FINANCIAL IMPLICATIONS OF CYSTIC FIBROSIS

Grants and benefits available in the United Kingdom in 1985

1. *Prescription Charges* No charge is made for any child under the age of 16 years. CF patients of 16 years or over, despite their continuing disability, are not entitled to an automatic exemption at the present time, but may purchase a four or 12 month prepaid 'season ticket' which covers the cost of all prescriptions. Leaflets are available at post offices and DHSS offices.

2. *Statutory Sick Pay and Sickness Benefit* These payments are made during relatively short periods of unemployment due to illness. If the person remains unable to work after a certain time has elapsed, they are replaced by the longer term *Invalidity Benefit*.

3. *Unemployment Benefit* This is paid to all people (CF or otherwise) who are unable to obtain employment, although capable of working. Certain National Insurance conditions have to be met.

4. *Supplementary Benefit* This is of particular relevance to older CF patients as it is payable to people aged 16 years or over who have little or no income and are unable to work because of continuing ill health. Certain expenses which have been incurred because of the illness itself (e.g. hospital outpatient visits) may also be paid.

5. *Family Income Supplement* A supplement is payable to families with children where the wage earner is in full-time employment

(defined as at least 30 hours per week for one of a couple and 24 hours for a single parent) and where the income is regarded as inadequate. This supplement bears no reference to whether any member of the family has CF. Leaflets may be obtained from DHSS offices.

6. *Attendance Allowance*   This grant is payable at two rates, and is available to children over the age of two years and adults who are severely disabled and need frequent attention 'in connection with bodily functions' by day, or both by day and by night. CF patients may qualify for the day allowance; it is unusual for them to qualify for the day and night allowance. Leaflets may be obtained from DHSS offices.

7. *Mobility Allowance*   This allowance is designed primarily for people over five years of age whose disability includes a specific difficulty in walking. Nevertheless CF patients with severe dyspnoea have been successful in obtaining this grant which may be used to assist with the expenses of running a car or for taxis or public transport.

8. *Other benefits*   which may be available in certain circumstances include free school meals, free milk and vitamins and exemption from dental and optical care. A comprehensive list can be found in leaflets entitled, 'Which Benefit?' and 'Help for Handicapped People' both available at DHSS offices.

9. *The Family Fund*   This charitable fund was set up to provide various different kinds of help for families who have severely handicapped children. It assists with the cost of equipment, transport, heating, structural alterations to the home and holidays. Further information is available from The Family Fund, PO Box 50, York, YO1 1UY, telephone number 0904–21115.

10. *The Cystic Fibrosis Research Trust*   operates a Holiday Caravan Scheme for affected children and their families. Well equipped caravans are located in suitable holiday areas in the United Kingdom, and can be rented. For information apply to the Executive Director, Cystic Fibrosis Research Trust, Alexandra House, 5 Blyth Road, Bromley, Kent BR1 3RS.

CARE OF THE DYING

Ultimately, repeated treatments and compensations fail, the usual cause of death being chronic obstructive respiratory disease and right heart failure.

The crucial observation on the part of the physician is to perceive when active treatments should cease (e.g. with antibiotics) and when palliative measures only should be taken.

During this time there are many drugs and treatments which can alleviate dyspnoea and the effects of sticky, infected secretions. Humidified oxygen, adequate hydration, sedation (chloral hydrate or diazepam, progressing to tincture of morphine or heroin, given on a regular basis) and antidepressants, all have their place. Physiotherapy should not be discontinued absolutely as gentle treatment can help to remove the secretions and more importantly, contact is maintained with a familiar figure.

It is of course vital that parents and other relatives should help with the care. Although some families prefer the patient to die in hospital, others request to take him home. The general practitioner and district nurse (visiting several times a day if needed) are able to provide adequate support and comfort for most cases. Domiciliary oxygen and suction apparatus can be supplied.

The hospital physician, general practitioner and social worker should always offer opportunities of talking with relatives after the death — not only immediately but during the months that follow. Sometimes comparative strangers can be helpful — the Society of Compassionate Friends, which aims to comfort bereaved parents by providing the companionship of other bereaved parents is one such organization (address: 6 Denmark Street, Bristol, BS1 5DQ, Telephone Number 0272–292778).

REFERENCES AND GENERAL READING

Allan JL, Townley RRW, Phelan PD. Family response to cystic fibrosis. *Aust Paediat J 1974; 10:* 136–146

Boyle IR, di Sant'Agnese PA, Sack S et al. Emotional adjustment of adolescents and young adults with cystic fibrosis. *J Pediatr 1976; 88:* 318–326

Brock DJH, Bedgood D, Barron L et al. Prospective prenatal diagnosis of cystic fibrosis. *Lancet 1985; i:* 1175–1178

Burton L, ed. *Care of the Child Facing Death.* London: Routledge and Kegan Paul. 1974

Burton L, ed. *The Family Life of Sick Children.* London: Routledge and Kegan Paul. 1975

Bywater EM. Adolescent with cystic fibrosis: psychosocial adjustment. *Arch Dis Childh 1981; 56:* 538–543

Bywater EM. Coping with a life-threatening illness: an experiment in parents' groups. *Br J Social Work 1984; 14:* 117–127

Chapman JA, Goodall J. Dying children need help too. *Br Med J 1979; 1:* 593–594

Cystic Fibrosis Research Trust Publications. 1) Lawson D. *Cystic Fibrosis.* 1981; 2) *Living with Cystic Fibrosis – A Guide for the Young Adult.* 1984; 3) Bentley B. *Attendance Allowance.* 1985; 4) *Problem? Who Can Help With What.* 1985

Drotar D, Doershuk CF, Stern RC et al. Psychosocial functioning of children with cystic fibrosis. *Pediatrics 1981; 67:* 338–343

Ellis CE, Hill E. Growth, intelligence and school performance in children with cystic fibrosis who have had an episode of malnutrition during infancy. *J Pediatr 1975; 87:* 565–568

Fagan E, Harwood I. Home care for the dying patient. In *Proceedings of the 8th International Congress of Cystic Fibrosis,Toronto, Canada.* Toronto: Canadian CF Foundation. 1980: 275–278

Falkman C. Cystic fibrosis – a psychological study of 52 children and their families. *Acta Paediatr Scand 1977; Suppl 269*

Harper PS. *Practical Genetic Counselling 2 Edn.* Bristol: John Wright and Sons Ltd. 1984

Lansdown R. *More Than Sympathy. The Everyday Needs of Sick and Handicapped Children and their Families.* London: Tavistock Publications. 1980

Lay Report and Report from 2nd International Cystic Fibrosis Adults Conference. *9th International CF Congress, Brighton.* Bromley: Cystic Fibrosis Trust. 1984

Lewis BL, Khaw K-T. Family functioning as a mediatory variable affecting psychosocial adjustment of children with cystic fibrosis. *J Pediatr 1982; 101:* 636–640

Lewiston NJ. Saturday's children: adolescents and adults with cystic fibrosis in today's society. *Proceedings of 8th International CF Congress, Toronto: Canada.* Toronto: Canadian CF Foundation. 1980: 266–274

Lewiston N, Conley J, Blessing-Moore J. Measurement of hypothetical burnout in cystic fibrosis caregivers. *Acta Paediatr Scand 1981; 70:* 935–939

McCollum AT, Gibson LE. Family adaptation to the child with cystic fibrosis. *J Pediat 1970; 77:* 571–578

McCrae WM. Psychological aspects of cystic fibrosis. In *Proceedings of the 11th Annual Meeting of the European Working Group for Cystic Fibrosis, Brussels.* Brussels: Belgian CF (M) Association. 1982: 11–17

McCrae WM, Cull AM, Burton et al. Cystic fibrosis: parents' response to the genetic basis of the disease. *Lancet 1973; ii:* 141–143

Michaud PA, Lasalle R, Frappier JY. The compliance of adolescents with cystic fibrosis. *Proceedings of 12th Annual Meeting EWGCF, Athens.* Athens: S Lennis. 1983: 253–258

Norman AP, Hodson ME. Emotional and social aspects of treatment. In Hodson ME, Norman AP, Batten JC, eds. *Cystic Fibrosis.* London: Bailliere Tindall. 1983: 242–259

Proceedings of the First International Cystic Fibrosis (Mucoviscidosis) Young Adults Meeting. Brussels. 1982

Rossi E, Buhlmann U, Kraemer R. Social and medical problems of cystic fibrosis in Switzerland. *Monogr Paediatr 1981; 14:* 192–201

Saunders CM. *The Management of Terminal Disease.* London: Arnold. 1978

Sinnema G, Bonarius JCJ, Stoop JW et al. Adolescents with cystic fibrosis in the Netherlands. *Acta Paediatr Scand 1983; 72:* 427–432

Stanghelle JK, Skyberg D. The successful completion of the Oslo Marathon by a patient with cystic fibrosis. *Acta Paediatr Scand 1983; 72:* 935–938

Strauss GD, Pedersen S, Dudovitz D. A psychosocial support for adults with cystic fibrosis. A group approach. *Am J Dis Child 1979; 133:* 301–305

Chapter 9

PROGNOSIS AND SCORING SYSTEMS

PROGNOSIS

During the early years of the recognition of cystic fibrosis, in the 1930s and 1940s, it was estimated that more than 80 per cent of the children afflicted died before their fifth birthday. Since then, and particularly since the 1960s, there has been a marked improvement — so much so that the best survival figures obtained from specialized 'CF Centres' have indicated that approximately 80 per cent should reach 19 or 20 years (Shwachman and Holsclaw, 1969, Boston, USA; Corey, 1980, Toronto, Canada; Phelan and Hey, 1984, Melbourne, Australia). Figures quoted from other CF centres are less good, but still impressive: an 80 per cent survival to 10–12 years and a 50 per cent survival to 20–22 years (Nielsen and Schiotz, 1982, Copenhagen, Denmark; Cystic Fibrosis Patient Registry, 1978, from several CF Centres in the USA and Canada).

For England and Wales, results have shown a similar trend: 80 per cent to 13–14 years, 70 per cent to 16 years for children attending the Hospital for Sick Children, London (Wilmott et al, 1983) and preliminary figures for *all* CF patients in England and Wales (whether attending a CF centre or not), 80 per cent to 13 years and 50 per cent to 20 years or more (BPA, 1985).

The reasons for this improvement in prognosis are complex, but four factors are considered relevant:

1. **earlier diagnosis and treatment;**

2. **development of more effective antibiotics;**

3. **the use of comprehensive and consistent treatment regimes;**

4. **the possibility that wider diagnosis reveals the existence of milder variants of the disease.**

The relative importance of each of these factors is uncertain but all may influence the future development of CF services. If earlier diagnosis profoundly affects the survival and quality of life (and this is not known with certainty) then newborn screening programmes are indicated. Alternatively, if particular treatment regimes are the most important factor, then many more controlled trials of standardized treatments are needed. If milder cases contribute substantially to the improvement in survival figures then this will complicate analysis of the results of any treatments used.

Several factors have an influence on *survival rates* in CF which *have been recorded in different ways and should be interpreted with care.*

The improving survival rate

Many studies, from different countries and different centres, demonstrate this change.

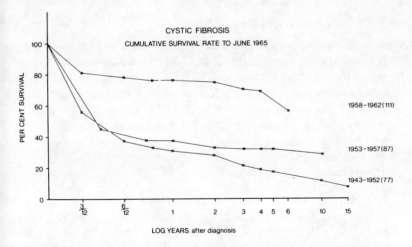

Figure 27. Cumulative survival rates from 1943 to 1962, of CF patients attending the Royal Children's Hospital, Melbourne, Australia. Graphs (logarithmic scale) constructed by CM Anderson (1967) and reproduced with permission

A survey of 275 CF children carried out in Melbourne in 1965 showed that of those diagnosed between 1943 and 1952, only 18 per cent were alive five years after diagnosis, while the corresponding figure for those diagnosed between 1958 and 1962 was 60 per cent (Figure 27). This result was attributed in part to earlier diagnosis and in part to more effective and consistent management (Anderson, 1967). Further notable improvements have occurred in Melbourne during the last 20 years, with 80 per cent survivals to 17 years (Phelan et al, 1979) and 20 years (Phelan and Hey, 1984).

A similar change was recorded in Philadelphia, where cumulative survival rates for patients diagnosed over three separate five year periods from 1952, were 35 per cent, 64 per cent and 77 per cent respectively (Huang et al, 1970).

Comparable improvements have been reported also from Sweden (Kollberg, 1982) and Denmark (Nielsen and Schiotz, 1982).

In London, England at the Hospital for Sick Children, a series of articles covers the years 1943 to 1979 (George and Norman, 1971; Robinson and Norman, 1975; Wilmott et al, 1983, Figure 28). While demonstrating the improved longevity overall, these papers give separate and detailed data on one of the factors which has affected survival — i.e. meconium ileus in the neonatal period.

The effect of meconium ileus

This presentation of CF, found in 10–15 per cent of CF babies during the first few days of life (see page 20) is treated by surgery in more than half the cases. Formerly (1943–1973) its presence had a substantial, although decreasing effect on survival figures. Wilmott et al (1983), reporting on figures for 1974 to 1979, has shown a marked improvement in survival figures for this group, much of it due to better survival in the first year (Figure 28a).

The influence of 'CF Centres'

Specialist CF clinics are now taking on much of the care of CF patients and fewer are attending their own paediatrician or chest physician exclusively. The arguments in favour of such centres include greater experience of the disease on the part of the physicians and health care team, and perhaps easier access to specialized physiotherapy and bacteriology services.

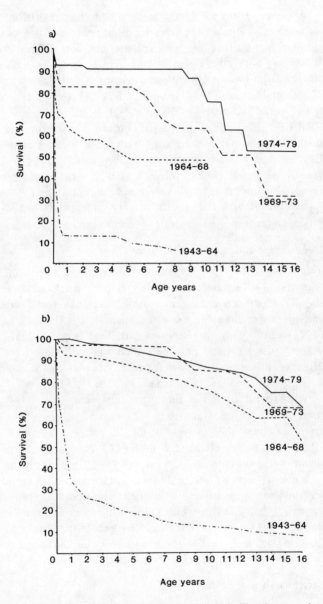

Figure 28 (a) and (b). Survival curves of children with cystic fibrosis, entered at birth: (a) meconium ileus patients, (b) non-meconium ileus patients. Reproduced from Wilmott et al, *Arch Dis Childh 1983; 38:* 835–836, with permission

Analyses of survival figures seem to be in favour of these centres — although care should be taken with interpretation of figures as some of the healthier patients (or their parents) may *seek* referral centre care. However this may be, Corey (1980) from Toronto, has reported better survival from the clinic there compared with Canada as a whole, as have Nielsen and Schiotz (1982) from the CF clinic in Copenhagen, compared with Denmark as a whole. Phelan and Hey (1984) considered that the total CF care provided at the CF Centre in Melbourne, was the chief reason for the better survival of patients in Victoria compared with England and Wales, where some are seen in CF clinics, and some in general paediatric clinics. Warwick (1982) has reviewed results from many CF clinics around the world and concludes that CF centre care, together with earlier diagnosis, are the principal factors which have produced the improved survivals of recent years.

Does the age at diagnosis affect survival?

This is not known precisely. Some observations suggest that it does. Warwick (1981) stated that, "analyses from the CF Patient Registry show that the average annual rate of death for children diagnosed early is lower than for those diagnosed late". George and Norman (1971) agreed with this. However, later data suggested that,"the value of early diagnosis will only be settled when neonatal screening with effective follow-up has been carried out in a co-ordinated manner over a wide region" (Robinson and Norman, 1975).

With regard to age *at diagnosis*, this seems to be fairly constant from several centres. Warwick (1982), observed that half the diagnoses are made during the first year of life, 90 per cent before 10 years and 99 per cent before 20 years. Kollberg (1982) recorded 50 per cent or slightly more during the first year and 75—80 per cent by three years.

Those patients who were diagnosed *much later than average* or who are surviving in good health in their late teens and early twenties, inevitably, must be those with milder symptoms. Duncan, Hodson and Batten (1981) who reported on 225 patients at the Brompton Hospital, London who had reached the age of 16 years, calculated that 46 per cent of these were likely to survive to 30 years.

Better survival of CF boys

This has been known for some time, although the difference is not great and apparent only on statistical analysis. Some workers have shown a

male survival somewhat greater than female, but only after 14 treatment years (Stern et al, 1976); others have found no significant difference
in a series of patients followed up to 16 years of age (Wilmott et al,
1983). By contrast, Nielsen and Schiotz (1982) recorded an excess
mortality of females over males at all ages up to 13 years of age, with
the exception of the first year.

No convincing explanation has been given for this phenomenon.

Other factors affecting survival

Extent of pulmonary damage on chest X-ray A study in Cleveland,
Ohio by Stern et al, 1976 has illustrated that the radiological score
of a chest X-ray, obtained one year after treatment, is a reliable guide
to survival. Patients were divided into two groups on this basis. Those
with minimal X-ray changes achieved a much better long-term survival
and a lower incidence of complications, than those with established
pulmonary disease.

Nutritional state It has long been suspected that a good nutritional
state is likely to be associated with better lung function and therefore,
with a better prognosis. Gaskin and his colleagues (1982) have been
able to study 48 CF patients who had a normal faecal fat excretion, in
comparison with CF patients who had the usual steatorrhoea. As a
group, the patients with a normal faecal fat were clinically milder, the
mean sweat chloride level was lower (although still within the CF range)
and pulmonary function tests showed less involvement.

Therefore a better prognosis is predicted for the group without
steatorrhoea. So far (1985), insufficient time has elapsed to verify
whether this is so.

QUALITY OF LIFE

The objective of management in CF is not only the prolongation of
life — this is not of supreme importance — it is the mitigation of the
extent to which the condition interferes with normal living.

Survival into young adult life and beyond is necessarily associated
with an increase in the complications of the disease, both medical and
psychological. Despite this, there have been several very encouraging
reports of the good quality of life which can be associated with longer
survival.

Seventy patients over the age of 25 years, treated at the Children's Hospital Medical Center, Boston, USA, achieved some outstanding successes (Shwachman, Kowalski and Khaw, 1977). Forty-one graduated from college, some following various professional careers which included physics, medicine, nursing, physiotherapy, teaching, law and engineering. Such a high proportion of professional qualifications illustrates the good intellect and considerable drive and ambition of these patients, referred to in an earlier chapter (Chapter 8). With regard to marriage and reproduction, 42 patients were married (24 males and 18 females). None of the males had fathered children although some couples had adopted; five women had one child each and one had two children.

More recent reports from Europe indicate a similar degree of motivation and achievement among adolescents and young adults. Among a very selected population of 316 patients over the age of 16 years who attended the Brompton Hospital, London, between 1965 and 1983 (Penketh, Wise, Mearns et al, 1985) 78 per cent were either in full-time education, full-time or part-time employment or were housewives, and only 13 per cent were unemployed on account of ill health. Thirteen per cent were married and ten women had borne children.

Associated with these improvements has been the growth of the *Association of CF Adults.* Patients themselves are coming together to discuss common problems, aspirations and achievements (page 197). Their positive attitude was summed up by the patient attending an International Conference who said, "Cystic Fibrosis is not a way of life; it is a part of life".

SCORING SYSTEMS

The varying manifestations and degrees of CF make it a difficult disease to evaluate, both in the individual and for a group. Some kind of system is necessary in order to assess a single patient and his need for treatment, to follow the development of the disease (e.g. after neonatal screening) and to monitor progress under different regimes of treatment.

Several systems have been devised. Some assess the patient as a whole, including some investigations, and others relate entirely to the changes seen on chest X-ray. The three scores of Shwachman and Kulczycki, Taussig et al and Cooperman et al are general assessments and those of Chrispin and Norman, and Brasfield et al, are radiological scores.

The Shwachman Score (Shwachman and Kulczycki, 1958)

This was one of the earliest schemes and is based on an assessment of four aspects: general activity, physical findings, nutritional status and chest X-ray appearances. A maximum of 25 points is given for each category and suggestions given for the allocation of points. A high score indicates a good clinical state, the gradings being 'excellent' (100—86), 'good' (85—71), 'mild' (70—56), 'moderate' (55—41) and 'severe' (40 and below).

Independent assessors who are familiar with the disease can achieve very similar scores for the same patient and such a system is useful in following the progress of individual patients. It is less valuable for comparing overall results between clinics.

This system has been modified by others, particularly to take into account the increasing age of the surviving patients and the increasing prevalence of complications, both of the respiratory tract and other affected organs such as the liver, pancreas and gastrointestinal tract.

The system of Taussig et al (1973)

This is simpler and permits assessment of the patient's past history, current status and prognosis and reflects any current situation more precisely. It is based predominantly upon pulmonary aspects as these mainly determine the prognosis. It emphasizes simple pulmonary function tests (implying of course, that the patient is old enough to perform such tests), utilizing vital capacity (VC), forced expiratory volume in one minute (FEV_1) as well as other features known to correlate with outlook: pneumothorax, haemoptysis, recent exacerbation of chest disease and cor pulmonale. Only a small proportion of points (25%) are related to body weight and activity. Attitude to the disease is considered to be important in older patients, as depression and 'adolescent rebellion' are associated frequently with deterioration in health.

Based on these scores the authors were able to construct a curve enabling a prediction to be made of the probability of death within three years — information which may not have great value in itself but which does suggest that the system is an accurate assessment of the clinical state and that it is reproducible.

The system of Cooperman et al (1971)

This test is probably the most straightforward to perform, but it has not been evaluated as fully as the preceding two tests.

The scoring system is based on five measurements:

(a)   general activity,

(b)   chest radiograph findings,

(c)   degree of finger clubbing,

(d)   growth and development,

(e)   complications.

Each feature is scored 2, 1 or 0. The sum of five individual scores is calculated (Table VIII). A patient in excellent health would have a score

TABLE VIII. Simplified CF scoring scale (after Cooperman et al 1971)

Dimensions for evaluation	Score		
	2	1	0
(a) *Activity*	Engages in athletics with normal peers Full activity	Attends regular school with normal peers – misses not more than 2 days per month	Any lesser performance
(b) *Chest X-ray*	Normal	Minimally increased markings and emphysema	Any worse features
(c) *Clubbing*	0 to 1+	1+ to 2+ with no cyanosis	2+ and greater
(d) *Growth and development*	Above 25th percentile for height and weight	Above 3rd percentile for height and weight	Below 3rd percentile for height and weight
(e) *Complications*	None	Transient	Fixed

Maximal total score of 10 reflects the best prognosis

of 10. Figure 29 illustrates serial scores to show progress. When discussing complications, the authors noted that a number of clinical features may be troublesome but they do not influence prognosis: these included rectal prolapse and nasal polyposis.

The final two systems are based on radiological findings.

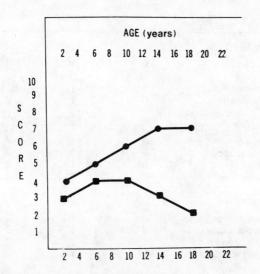

Figure 29. Scoring system of Cooperman et al (1971). Graphs of the progress of two patients during an 18 year follow-up, one patient showing improvement and the other deterioration. Total scores were entered yearly at the time of the annual X-ray of the chest

The radiological score of Chrispin and Norman (1974)

Antero-posterior and lateral chest radiographs are viewed jointly by two observers in order to reduce observer error to a minimum and to achieve agreement on the severity of the changes. Abnormalities are scored on a scale of 0–2, the four quadrants of the lung fields being assessed independently. In addition, changes in chest configuration are noted and scored on a similar scale (Table IX). A high score (maximum 38 points, see Table IX) indicates a poor chest X-ray.

Bronchial line shadows are those which appear to be due to prominence of the bronchial shadows. Mottled shadows are multiple small rounded shadows with rather ill-defined edges measuring up to 0.5cm

TABLE IX.   X-ray evaluation by the scoring system of Chrispin and Norman
(1974). Radiographic features and points awarded according to severity.
(Reproduced from Chrispin and Norman. *Pediat Radiol 1974; 2:* 101–106,
with permission)

Feature	Not present	Present but not marked	Marked
Chest configuration:			
Sternal bowing	0	1	2
Diaphragmatic			
depression	0	1	2
Spinal kyphosis	0	1	2
Bronchial line shadows:			
Right upper zone	0	1	2
Right lower zone	0	1	2
Left upper zone	0	1	2
Left lower zone	0	1	2
Mottled shadows:			
Right upper zone	0	1	2
Right lower zone	0	1	2
Left upper zone	0	1	2
Left lower zone	0	1	2
Ring shadows:			
Right upper zone	0	1	2
Right lower zone	0	1	2
Left upper zone	0	1	2
Left lower zone	0	1	2
Large shadows:			
Right upper zone	0	1	2
Right lower zone	0	1	2
Left upper zone	0	1	2
Left lower zone	0	1	2

in diameter. *Ring shadows* which are formed by a central area of
increased lung translucency clearly circumscribed by a discrete outline,
are commonly 0.5cm in diameter and seen predominantly in the peri-
phery. *Large shadows* are caused by confluent areas of collapse/consoli-
dation affecting a lobe or a segment.

The system provides a reproducible method of scoring serial X-rays and a high degree of inter-observer agreement has been found. It has been shown to correlate well with changes of lung function (Matthew et al, 1977).

The radiological score of Brasfield et al (1979)

This system is similar to that of Chrispin and Norman but uses a wider scale of severity (0–4) and measures changes in the lung fields as a whole rather than by region. The maximum total score is 25 and points are deducted for abnormalities; thus a high score in this case indicates a good chest X-ray. Five categories are measured: *air trapping, linear markings, nodular-cystic lesions, large lesions* (this includes an additional point for multiple atelectasis) and *general severity* (this also includes another point for such complications as cardiomegaly and pneumothorax).

Brasfield's system has also been found to have a high degree of reproducibility by and between observers. It also correlates well with the results of pulmonary function tests and the X-ray component of the Shwachman score (for this reason a total of 25 points was allocated as this is the total number given to the chest X-ray component of the Shwachman score).

An independent comparison of the Shwachman, Chrispin-Norman and Brasfield systems has shown none to be markedly better than the others (Dankert-Roelse et al, 1984).

REFERENCES AND GENERAL READING

Prognosis and survival

Anderson CM. Long-term study of patients with cystic fibrosis. *Mod Probl Pediatr 1967; 10:* 344–349

Barbero GJ. Commentary: the clinical forms of cystic fibrosis. *J Pediatr 1982; 100:* 914–915

BPA. *British Paediatric Association Working Group on Cystic Fibrosis.* 1985. Unpublished report

Corey ML. Longitudinal studies in cystic fibrosis. In Sturgess JM, ed. *Perspectives in Cystic Fibrosis. Proceedings of the 8th International CF Congress, Toronto, Canada.* Toronto: Canadian CF Foundation. 1980: 246

Cystic Fibrosis Foundation: Report of the Patient Registry. Vol 1978. Rockville, Maryland: CF Foundation. 1980

Duncan FR, Hodson ME, Batten JC. Cystic Fibrosis – survival into adult life. *Eur J Pediatr 1981; 137:* 125

Editorial. Survival in cystic fibrosis. *Lancet 1984; i:* 663–664

Gaskin K, Gurwitz D, Durie P et al. Improved respiratory diagnosis in CF patients with normal fat absorption. *J Pediatr 1982; 100:* 857–862

George L, Norman AP. Life tables for cystic fibrosis. *Arch Dis Childh 1971; 46:* 139–143

Gurwitz D, Corey M, Francis PWJ et al. Perspectives in cystic fibrosis. *Pediatr Clin North Am 1979; 26:* 603–615

Huang NN, Macri CN, Girone J et al. Survival of patients with cystic fibrosis. *Am J Dis Child 1970; 120:* 289–295

Kollberg H. Incidence and survival curves of cystic fibrosis in Sweden. *Acta Paediatr Scand 1982; 71:* 197–202

Nielsen OH, Schiotz PO. Cystic fibrosis in Denmark in the period 1945–1981. Evaluation of centralized treatment. *Acta Paediatr Scand 1982; Suppl 301:* 107–119

Phelan PD, Allan JL, Landau LI et al. Improved survival of patients with cystic fibrosis. *Med J Aust 1979; 1:* 261–263

Phelan PD, Hey E. Cystic fibrosis mortality in England and Wales and in Victoria, Australia, 1976–1980. *Arch Dis Childh 1984; 59:* 71–83

Robinson MJ, Norman AP. Life tables for cystic fibrosis. *Arch Dis Childh 1975; 50:* 962–965

Shwachman H, Holsclaw DS. Complications of cystic fibrosis. *N Engl J Med 1969; 281:* 500–501

Stern RC, Boat TF, Doershuk CF et al. Course of cystic fibrosis in 95 patients. *J Pediatr 1976; 89:* 406–411

Warwick WJ. The natural history of cystic fibrosis. In Warwick WJ, ed. *1000 Years of Cystic Fibrosis*. Minnesota: University of Minnesota. 1981: 13–27

Warwick WJ. Prognosis for survival with cystic fibrosis: the effects of early diagnosis and cystic fibrosis center care. *Acta Paediatr Scand 1982; Suppl 301:* 27–31

Wilcken B, Towns SJ, Mellis CM. Diagnostic delay in cystic fibrosis: lessons from newborn screening. *Arch Dis Childh 1983; 58:* 863–866

Wilmott RW, Tyson SL, Dinwiddie R et al. Survival rates in cystic fibrosis. *Arch Dis Childh 1983; 58:* 835–838

Quality of life

di Sant'Agnese PA, Davis PB. Cystic fibrosis in adults. Seventy-five cases and a review of 232 cases in the literature. *Am J Med 1979; 66:* 121–132

Penketh ARL, Wise A, Mearns MB et al. Cystic fibrosis in adolescents and adults. *Thorax 1985.* In press

Shwachman H, Kowalski M, Khaw K-T. Cystic fibrosis: a new outlook. Seventy patients above 25 years of age. *Medicine 1977; 56:* 129–149

Scoring Systems

Brasfield D, Hicks G, Soong S-J et al. The chest roentgenogram in cystic fibrosis: a new scoring system. *Pediatrics 1979; 63:* 24–29

Chrispin AR, Norman AP. The systematic evaluation of the chest radiograph in cystic fibrosis. *Pediat Radiol 1974; 2:* 101–106

Coates AL, Boyce P, Shaw DG et al. Relationship between chest radiograph, regional lung function studies, exercise tolerance, and clinical condition in cystic fibrosis. *Arch Dis Childh 1981; 56:* 106–111

Cooperman EM, Park M, McKee J et al. A simplified cystic fibrosis scoring system. *Canad Med Ass J 1971; 105:* 580–582

Dankert-Roelse JE, Martijn A, te Meerman GJ et al. A comparison of the Shwachman, Chrispin-Norman and Brasfield method for scoring of chest radiographs of patients with cystic fibrosis. In Lawson D, ed. *Cystic Fibrosis Horizons. Proceedings of the 9th International CF Congress, Brighton.* Chichester: John Wiley and Sons. 1984: 264

Mathew DJ, Warner JO, Chrispin AR et al. The relationship between chest radiographic scores and respiratory function tests in children with cystic fibrosis. *Pediatr Radiol 1977; 5:* 198–200

Shwachman H, Kulczycki LL. Long-term study of 105 patients with cystic fibrosis. *Am J Dis Child 1958; 96:* 6–15

Taussig LM, Kattwinkel J, Friedewald WT et al. A new prognostic score and clinical evaluation system for cystic fibrosis. *J Pediatr 1973: 82:* 380–390

Chapter 10

LABORATORY INVESTIGATIONS

In this chapter, the nature of each test and the indication for its use will be discussed, but actual techniques will be given only in outline. These details may be obtained from the references listed at the end of the chapter.

THE SWEAT TEST

Abnormally high concentrations of sodium and chloride in the sweat of patients with cystic fibrosis were first reported in 1953 by di Sant'Agnese and his colleagues. The abnormality is present from birth. It is found in at least 98 per cent of individuals with cystic fibrosis and in only a very few other well-defined conditions such as adrenal cortical insufficiency, ectodermal dysplasia and rare genetic metabolic defects - all capable of precise diagnosis and unlikely to be mistaken for CF. **The sweat test is therefore the essential investigation for the diagnosis of cystic fibrosis** and should be viewed in conjunction with the history, clinical and radiological findings and ancillary biochemical tests. It is imperative that it should be as accurate, precise and reliable as modern laboratory methods can make it.

A number of techniques have been used, both for stimulating and collecting sweat and for estimating its electrolyte content.

The *standard procedure,* in which sweating is stimulated by pilocarpine iontophoresis, followed by analysis of the sweat to determine its sodium and chloride content, was described by Gibson and Cooke (1959).

Older methods of sweat collection, such as enclosing a limb in a plastic bag, should not be used for diagnostic purposes, as electrolyte levels although elevated, have a different range from those in sweat produced by pilocarpine iontophoresis. In addition, severe salt losses can occur.

Rapid estimations of sweat electrolytes by ion-specific electrodes applied directly to the skin, or by machines to measure conductivity, are not sufficiently reliable for routine use (Kopito and Shwachman, 1968; Bray et al, 1977; Denning et al, 1980).

More recent systems for sweat collection, with the use of a heated cup, or capillary tubing and measurement of osmolality (see page 164) show good results but so far they have not replaced the standard method as the definitive sweat test for cystic fibrosis.

Pilocarpine iontophoresis method (Gibson and Cooke, 1959)

Pilocarpine stimulates autonomic effector cells. Although the drug can penetrate the intact skin, percutaneous transfer is enhanced by iontophoresis, in which a small electric current is passed through a solution of the drug applied to the skin. This produces a local concentration of pilocarpine which stimulates the sweat glands, but without systemic effects.

The test consists of two parts:

1. *accurate collection of at least 100mg of uncontaminated sweat;*

2. *laboratory estimation of sodium and chloride.*

It must be performed with meticulous attention to detail. Usually, in any one hospital, the sweat test is carried out by only one or two people. It is not a procedure for the casual operator.

Personnel concerned should have established their own values in controls and should perform the tests sufficiently often to maintain expertise. **If these criteria cannot be met, it is best to refer the patient to a larger paediatric or CF centre where the test is done regularly.**

It should always be repeated if the result, clinical features and stool microscopy/faecal fat excretion are not in agreement. If the sweat test is inconclusive all the clinical and investigatory evidence must be carefully reviewed.

The test involves the patient for about 40 minutes, is not painful or inconvenient and can be used with safety in very young, small or moderately ill babies (in very ill babies the test may give an erroneous result).

Collection of sweat This is the most difficult part of the test, that is, the part most subject to error. A nurse or laboratory technician with special training is a much more appropriate person to collect the sweat than an inexperienced doctor.

1. The area preferred for stimulation of sweating is the forearm, but in thin or small babies the thigh or even the back may be used.

2. The flexor surface of the forearm is washed with distilled water and dried with gauze.

3. The positive electrode is covered with four layers of absorbent lint, BPC. This pad of lint is then soaked in 0.4 per cent pilocarpine nitrate solution and placed, lint downwards, on the washed skin surface.

4. The negative electrode is also covered with four layers of absorbent lint but this pad is soaked with N/10 magnesium sulphate solution (or one per cent potassium hypophosphate, K_2HPO_4). The damp surface is applied to the extensor surface of the same arm, or the opposite arm. Both electrodes are secured with stockinette bandaging.

5. Care should be taken that no part of the metal electrodes is in contact with the skin, otherwise a slight burn may occur when the current is passed.

6. Turn on the current and increase gradually to 4ma, which is then applied for five minutes.

7. Remove the electrodes. Wash the skin where the pilocarpine was iontophoresed, with distilled water and dry with ethanol. This area, from which the sweat is now to be collected, must be quite dry and free from any contamination (e.g. baby powder or antiseptic).

8. Using forceps, a dry, preweighed filter paper is removed from its covered container (stoppered flask or petri dish) and placed on the iontophoresed skin. The paper is completely covered with polythene or 'cling film', making sure that there is an air-tight seal (using masking tape if necessary). A crepe bandage is put on to keep everything in

place and keep the arm warm. A cardigan may also be brought down over the arm, for warmth and to prevent the child interfering with the bandage.

9. After at least 20 minutes, the filter paper which is now soaked with sweat, is removed with forceps and transferred back into the covered container (to avoid evaporation). The container is reweighed.

At least 100mg of sweat is necessary.

10. The sweat is eluted with 5ml of distilled water.

There are a number of minor variations to the above technique − in particular some operators do not cover the electrodes with absorbent lint, relying on filter papers alone but we feel that the lint prevents the possibility of a small burn. We also prefer not to use saline under the negative electrode. In the case of small babies it is sometimes necesary to stimulate sweat in two places and elute both filter papers together, to obtain enough sweat.

Some practical clinical points *Dehydration* should be repaired before the test is done. Areas of *oedema* can produce reduced sweat levels. *Repeated stimulation* over the same area can cause exhaustion of glands, with an increase in electrolyte concentrations.

Laboratory estimation of sodium and chloride Micromethods are needed. Sodium concentrations are usually estimated by flame photometry and chloride by titration.

Results are expressed as mmol/L. Values should be given for *both* sodium *and* chloride, and for the weight of sweat.

Interpretation of the sweat test and normal values

The majority of young children have sweat sodium and chloride concentrations below 40mmol/L and in the first years of life they may be as low as 10−15mmol/L. If values are between 50 and 60mmol/L the test should be repeated and if still in the same range, should be considered carefully together with the other evidence before a decision is made about the diagnosis. This applies to values between 40 and 60 mmol/L in babies less than one year of age.

Concentrations of both ions above 60mmol/L should definitely be considered abnormal in childhood.

Values for sodium and chloride should not differ widely — a discrepancy of more than 15mmol/L in the lower ranges increasing to 30 mmol/L in the higher, is an indication for a repeat test.

Sweat concentrations *greater than normal serum levels* are also suspect and the test should be repeated.

Potassium concentrations are slightly raised in CF sweat (Shwachman, Mahmoodian and Neff, 1981) and may account for some of the difference between chloride and sodium levels (chloride levels tend to be higher than sodium in CF patients, whereas these values are usually equal in controls).

Normal infants may show borderline, or raised sweat test values during the first few days of life (Hardy et al, 1973). It is partly for this reason that the sweat test is not usually done during the first week after birth. (Another, and equally important reason is the difficulty in obtaining sufficient sweat at this time).

Values in children with cystic fibrosis

Values over 60mmol/L should be considered abnormal. The majority lie between 80 and 125mmol/L.

Shwachman et al (1981) who studied 252 CF children in comparison with 252 controls, found mean values in the CF patients, for sodium, chloride and potassium to be 111, 115 and 23mmol/L respectively, whereas the corresponding figures for the control subjects, were 28, 28 and 10mmol/L, respectively.

It is thought that less than two per cent of CF patients have values between 50 and 60mmol/L and that perhaps 1:1000 have values near the upper limit of the 'normal range', that is, below 50mmol/L (di Sant'Agnese, 1981).

Sweat electrolytes in adolescents and adults

Unfortunately the sweat test is less discriminating after puberty, as sweat electrolyte levels tend to rise with age and values in non-CF people may reach 60–90mmol/L (Anderson and Freeman, 1960; McKendrick, 1962).

When making a diagnosis of CF in an adult, it has been suggested that at least *two* sweat *sodium* values of more than 70mmol/L should be obtained on separate occasions (Hodson et al, 1983). All other clinical and investigatory evidence should be considered carefully as well (see page 43).

Pretreatment with fludrocortisone increases the diagnostic usefulness of the sweat test in adults. After a baseline sweat test has been done, on day one, a daily dose of $3mg/m^2$ of 9-alpha-fluorohydrocortisone is given for two days. Repeat sweat tests on days four and five show a substantial depression of sodium concentrations in the majority of normal adults (mean value 26%) and a much smaller depression, or none at all, in the CF patients (mean value 9%) (Hodson et al, 1983).

Sweat electrolytes in parents and siblings

Sweat test values in known heterozygotes (i.e. the parents of CF people) are very little different from those of normal controls. When large numbers are tested, heterozygotes show a marginal increase compared with the population at large, *but the test is of no value in detecting individual carriers.*

Some two-thirds of the siblings of CF patients (statistically, see page 6) will be heterozygotes for CF, *but they cannot be distinguished on the basis of a sweat test.*

However, in the absence of clinical symptoms, in the vast majority of cases, the sweat test can be used quite satisfactorily to exclude the diagnosis of CF (the *homozygous* state) in the siblings.

Other conditions in which elevated sweat electrolytes have been found

None of these should cause difficulty in differential diagnosis and include:

> adrenal insufficiency,
> ectodermal dysplasia,
> familial hypoparathyroidism,
> hypothyroidism,
> glucose-6-phosphatase deficiency,
> pitressin-resistant diabetes insipidus,
> nephrosis,

severe malnutrition,
fucosidosis,
glycogen storage disease, type 1,
mucopolysaccharidoses,
Mauriac's syndrome,
familial cholestasis syndrome.

'Normal' sweat electrolytes in cystic fibrosis

The 'grey area' of sweat electrolyte values (50–60mmol/L in children) can cause problems with diagnosis, which must remain in doubt unless there is strong supportive clinical evidence. Nevertheless, there are now several reports of patients with borderline sweat values (representing less than two per cent of the total CF population) whose symptoms of respiratory infection, often with pancreatic disorder, are highly suggestive of CF (Shwachman et al, 1966; Cogswell, Risdon and Taylor, 1974; Sarsfield and Davies 1975; Schwarz, Simpson and Ahuja, 1977; Stern et al, 1978; Editorial 1978; Huff, Huang and Arey, 1979; Davis, Hubbard and di Sant'Agnese, 1980; Collins and Rolles, 1985).

Suggestions that some of these patients may represent genetic variants of CF (Stern et al, 1978) are not proven. There is data to show that patients with normal pancreatic function tend to have lower values for sweat electrolytes (Davis et al, 1980).

Modifications of the standard sweat test

Measurement of *sweat osmolality* is gaining acceptance for the diagnosis of CF. Satisfactory correlations have been found between these values and sweat sodium concentrations and at least two groups have reported no overlap between CF and normal values (Carter et al, 1984; Schoni et al, 1984). The techniques can be used on babies in the first weeks of life.

Systems incorporate pilocarpine iontophoresis and sweat is collected either into a heated cup (Webster and Barlow, 1981; Kirk et al, 1983; Schoni et al, 1984) to eliminate condensation and evaporation, or, more effectively, into capillary tubing (Macroduct system, ChemLab Instruments Ltd) which can be sealed after collection (Carter et al, 1984). Osmolality measurements are made on eight microlitre samples using a vapour pressure osmometer (Wescor, ChemLab Instruments Ltd).

Other devices have been made for office and clinic use (Medtronic Screening System) and are recommended for *screening only* (see page 172) prior to the performance of a formal sweat test (Warwick et al, 1983).

Pitfalls in the diagnosis of cystic fibrosis

Difficulties in diagnosis relate to at least three areas:

1. choice of sweat test;

2. the test itself;

3. correlation of sweat test values with other laboratory and clinical features.

There is no doubt that the disease has been both overdiagnosed (Smalley, Addey and Anderson, 1978; David and Phillips, 1982) and underdiagnosed (Wilcken, Towns and Mellis, 1983). Inappropriate sweat test methods, such as the use of the chloride electrode and conductivity tests for *diagnosis rather than for screening,* have contributed to these difficulties.

TESTS FOR EXOCRINE PANCREATIC INSUFFICIENCY

Most patients with CF have marked steatorrhoea. Demonstration of its presence helps to confirm the diagnosis, and is essential before instituting pancreatic replacement therapy.

Fat globules in stools

Stools contain a large amount of unsplit fat, evident as oily droplets on stool microscopy. Their demonstration is a simple procedure which can be readily performed in the clinic or ward side-room provided a microscope is available. A sample of fresh stool is mixed with a drop of water on a glass slide to make a thin film which is examined under a cover slip with or without staining. *Numerous oily droplets are seen in each high power field* (Figure 8, page 33). Droplets are spherical, vary in size and are slightly refractile. They float to the surface of the preparation and therefore come into focus before the depth of the slide is reached — and are best seen by focusing up and down. Of course, they will only be present if the diet contains fat.

Other conditions in which similar findings occur include:

acute gastroenteritis in a child still taking milk;
obstructive jaundice;
other forms of pancreatic insufficiency (e.g. Shwachman-Diamond syndrome).

Oil used for lubricating a rectal thermometer may cause error. In coeliac disease only very occasional fat globules are seen as fat usually appears as fatty acid crystals or soapy masses. Premature babies may show a few fat globules in the stools.

Value of test Stool examination by microscopy is useful as a preliminary test when considering an infant with persistent cough or recurrent bronchitis. A negative result should not defer further examination by sweat test if there is clinical suspicion of CF, but a positive result may be helpful. The test is also useful in assessment of a new sibling in the family, because it may be positive within 48 hours of the introduction of milk feeds, well before a sweat test may be possible. It may also be used as an initial follow up to a positive screening test (see page 170).

Definitely positive tests will denote steatorrhoea due to pancreatic insufficiency and no further tests for malabsorption or pancreatic function are necessary in most cases.

A negative test in the presence of a positive sweat test will indicate the need for measurement of fat excretion in a stool collection and perhaps for other tests of pancreatic function.

After infancy the examination of the stool may also reveal some meat fibres and many undigested starch grains which stain blue when iodine is added to the stool.

Faecal fat assay

Analysis of the total fat content of a three-day collection of stools will confirm the presence and severity of steatorrhoea, provided that the patient's dietary fat intake is adequate. An infant should receive 3g of fat per kg body weight, and older children and adults 30—100g per day, according to body weight. (For methodology see Anderson, Burke and Gracey, 1986).

Normal stools contain no more than 5g of fat per day, whereas CF stools often contain 15–30g per day, the coefficient of absorption being 50 per cent or less.

It is important that those CF patients who have a normal faecal fat excretion should be recognized as they do not require pancreatic enzyme therapy. This is not only wasteful but can produce faecal masses and abdominal pain simulating the 'meconium ileus equivalent' syndrome.

Tests of pancreatic enzymes

Standard tests for the assessment of pancreatic function are the pancreozymin-secretin test (Hadorn et al, 1968) and the Lundh meal (Bergstrom and Lundh, 1970; McCollum, Muller and Harries, 1977). Both of these require duodenal intubation, but it is not necessary to carry out such a test on each CF child. If clinical features are suggestive and steatorrhoea present, the sweat test is sufficient confirmation of the disease. However, there are clinical situations when further studies of pancreatic function are necessary:

1. *when the result of the sweat test is persistently equivocal or is normal, but other features strongly suggest the disease;*

2. *in patients presenting for the first time during adolescence or adult life and sweat electrolyte levels are over 60mmol/L;*

3. *in the 10–15 per cent of patients who have normal stools.*

In some cases, intubation may be avoided with the use of the PABA test (see below).

Pancreozymin-secretin test After an overnight fast, and under sedation and fluoroscopic control, both the duodenum and stomach are intubated and attached to continuous suction pumps. Collections are made, at timed intervals, of the fasting duodenal juice, followed by the samples produced in response to the slow intravenous injections of pancreozymin-cholecystokinin, one to two units per kg and secretin, two units per kg. Analyses of trypsin, lipase, amylase and bicarbonate concentrations are then carried out in the laboratory (Anderson, Burke and Gracey, 1986).

The vast majority of CF patients will show abnormalities by this test, even those who have a normal faecal fat excretion. In this group, *enzyme concentrations* may be normal, but duodenal juice will be mucoid, of small volume and show a negligible increase in volume or rise in bicarbonate content after stimulation with secretin.

Lundh meal This relies upon the stimulatory effects of a standard meal to produce a pancreatic exocrine response. The meal used in children consists of carbohydrate (4%) in the form of glucose, protein (4%) as comminuted chicken and fat (4%) as corn oil. The dosage is 30ml/kg body weight up to a maximum of 240ml.

After an overnight fast, and sedation, a collecting tube is passed into the fourth part of the duodenum and a nasogastric tube for the administration of the meal. A baseline aspiration for 30 minutes is obtained before the meal is given and subsequent collections may be either as 20 minute aliquots or as a pooled two hour aspiration. The fluid is analysed for enzyme activity. Children with cystic fibrosis have shown marked reductions in duodenal fluid enzyme concentrations (trypsin, lipase and esterase).

The PABA test The synthetic peptide N-benzoyl-L-tyrosyl para-aminobenzoic acid (PABA peptide) is cleaved by pancreatic chymotrypsin in the duodenum and the PABA released is absorbed via the gut and excreted in the urine. This gives an indirect measure of chymotrypsin activity and has the advantage of being non-invasive. It is of course important that children having the test should not be taking pancreatic enzyme supplements at the time.

The patient should be fasted overnight, and an oral dose of PABA peptide is given in the morning. Doses which we have found adequate have been 500mg for adults and 8mg/kg body weight for children. Overnight urine is discarded and a urine collection made for the next six hours. This is tested for its PABA content.

Good separations have been found between values for controls (57–79% of the ingested PABA dose) and CF patients with pancreatic enzyme insufficiency (1–6%) (Custance et al, 1981). Some workers have shown a good correlation between PABA recovery and the degree of steatorrhoea (Nousia-Arvantitakis et al, 1978) while others have not (Bravo et al, 1983). It is not suitable for use in infants younger than five months, in whom a considerable overlap between CF and control results is seen (Sacher, Kobsa and Shmerling, 1978).

This test has been well validated and if it is abnormal it is not usually necessary to proceed to further documentation of pancreatic enzyme insufficiency.

If malabsorption from coeliac disease or some other defect of mucosal uptake of PABA is suspected, a preliminary investigation using oral PABA without the peptide should be carried out on the previous day. In uncomplicated CF absorption of PABA itself will be normal and a significant difference between urinary excretion of absorbed PABA and PABA peptide will indicate chymotrypsin deficiency.

Serum levels of PABA can also be measured, so avoiding the collection of urine specimens (Dockter, Nacu, Kohlberger, 1981).

A similar tubeless test, measuring esterase activity against fluorescein dilaurate has been described but has not been evaluated in CF (Barry et al, 1982).

Serum immunoreactive trypsin (IRT) The serum trypsin test is not an ideal guide to pancreatic exocrine function and is mainly useful for neonatal screening (page 171). However, when pancreatic damage has progressed to the point where enzyme secretion ceases, serum levels are very low or unrecordable (Dandona et al, 1979). On the other hand, normal or elevated serum trypsin levels give no indication of the adequacy or otherwise of the pancreatic secretions reaching the duodenum.

Other tests for malabsorption

A number of other tests can be used to demonstrate malabsorption due to pancreatic insufficiency, e.g. *stool trypsin or chymotrypsin* (Bonin et al, 1973). Perhaps the simplest test for routine use is the measurement of *serum triglycerides and/or chylomicrons* after a fatty meal (Fallstrom, Nygren and Olegard, 1977; Goldstein et al, 1983). Absorption of ^{14}C triglycerides and fatty acids can be measured indirectly by the *concentration of $^{14}CO_2$ in the breath,* but this is not uniformly reliable and should not be used as a routine.

Serum estimations of isoamylases show reduced levels of *pancreatic amylase* (Taussig et al, 1974; Skude and Kollberg, 1976; Kenny et al, 1978; Gillard et al, 1984) and in some cases, *increased* levels of salivary amylase. Low concentrations have been found for *pancreatic lipase* activity (Junglee et al, 1983).

NEONATAL SCREENING

The identification of various diseases in the newborn infant (phenyl-ketonuria, hypothyroidism) by means of blood tests, has been in operation for some time, but there is no agreement on whether such tests should be applied to the identification of CF infants. Some feel that potential benefits may not be sufficient for screening to be carried out on a general population basis (Committee Report, 1983; Holtzman, 1984) while others are more optimistic (Dodge and Ryley, 1982; Editorial, 1984; Farrell, 1984).

The ideal test would be one which is cheap, painless, simple, *specific to CF* (that is no babies would be identified as having CF when they do not) and *sensitive* (that is it would detect all cases).

No such ideal test exists and those which have been used have certain disadvantages.

It has been proposed that the screening for a disease on a national scale is justified if the following criteria apply (Wilson and Jungner, 1968).

1. The disease is an important health problem for the individual and the community.

2. Its natural history is known.

3. It has a latent or early symptomatic state.

4. It can be identified by a suitable screening test.

5. The facilities for definitive diagnosis and treatment are available and treatment policy is agreed.

6. The natural history of the disease is favourably modified by early, acceptable treatment.

7. The exercise is cost-effective.

Not all these criteria have been met in the case of cystic fibrosis — in particular more information is needed on items 5 and 6. Nevertheless, with the advent of a satisfactory blood test for neonatal screening (Crossley, Elliott and Smith, 1979), the opportunity has presented for an assessment of the value of screening, using blood spots already obtained for the screening of other diseases. Screening studies are being pursued in limited areas, with careful clinical follow up of infants ascertained as having CF.

It remains to be shown that identification of presymptomatic infants with CF is justifiable. It is of course essential that such babies should be given appropriate treatment and that this should be maintained if any benefit is to be expected. Because of the very variable course of the disease, it will be necessary to follow up substantial numbers of such babies and compare their progress with that of children diagnosed after clinical presentation, in order to answer this fundamental question.

Preliminary reports suggest that the outcome for babies detected by screening is more favourable than for those recognized by symptoms (Dankert-Roelse et al, 1983; Mastella et al, 1983). Further studies and longer follow up are required.

Methods for neonatal screening

1. Immunoreactive trypsin (or trypsinogen) test (IRT) The measurement of this enzyme, in serum or in blood, is the most appropriate and reliable test for neonatal screening and *is independent of the amount of residual pancreatic function.*

Serum IRT is five or ten times higher in the blood of newborn infants with CF compared with healthy neonates (Crossley, Elliott and Smith, 1979). Levels remain high up to the ages of two to six months, after which they fall. *The mechanism* for this high level of IRT in the CF baby is thought to be a partial blockage of the pancreatic duct, with 'back leakage' of the acinar contents into the plasma.

Commercial kits for the measurement of serum IRT are available from at least two companies (Hoechst, CIS) and assays can be adapted to measure IRT in the dried *blood* spots which are obtained from all babies on the seventh to tenth days of life, for the detection of phenylketonuria and hypothyroidism.

The test is considerably more specific than the meconium screening tests; false positive results can be reduced to about 0.45 per cent with experience. Again in comparison with the meconium tests, false negative results are fewer, being less than five per cent (with the exception of babies with meconium ileus, where for some unknown reason, false negative tests are not common – Duhamel et al, 1984).

It is difficult to calculate cost-effectiveness, but the current cost of an IRT test, excluding technician's salary, is about 40p per test, or £800 per patient diagnosed.

A similar test for the measurement of immunoreactive pancreatic lipase has been proposed (Hammond, Ask and Watts, 1984). This may be useful for reducing the number of false positive IRT results.

2. Meconium test The detection of CF by means of meconium analysis depends on the recognition of undigested protein (albumin) which is secondary to pancreatic enzyme insufficiency. Normal meconium contains less than 0.1mg albumin/g of meconium; CF meconium, when the patient has pancreatic dysfunction, contains an average of 200mg/g.

The increased albumin can be measured semiquantitatively by a test strip method (BM sticks, produced by Boehringer Mannheim) but unfortunately, as would be expected, up to 30 per cent of specimens give a false negative result. False positive results are about 0.5 per cent in full-term infants and greater in the premature or in the presence of gastrointestinal bleeding. The false positive incidence can be reduced by various additional tests such as the measurement of lactase (Antonowicz, Ishida and Shwachman, 1976; Berry, Kellogg and Lichstein, 1980) or of the albumin:alpha$_1$ trypsin inhibitor ratio (Ryley et al, 1979).

There is currently no screening test on meconium which can be recommended.

3. Faeces test This test, based on an assay of trypsin or chymotrypsin, is also dependent on pancreatic function and has a similar incidence of false negatives and false positive results as the meconium test. Although it can be carried out on faecal material smeared on cards, which simplifies despatch, it is not a suitable test for screening for CF.

4. Other approaches None is satisfactory. The sweat test, as performed by pilocarpine iontophoresis, is obviously too time-consuming and complicated for routine use. *Chloride ion electrodes* applied directly to the skin have been used but they are unreliable in practice.

It should be emphasized that the above tests are *screening tests* only, and that a positive result, even by serum or blood IRT, should be followed by a second screening test, and a standard pilocarpine iontophoresis sweat test, before a diagnosis of cystic fibrosis is made.

RESPIRATORY FUNCTION TESTS

These tests do not assist in the diagnosis of CF but are used to assess progress and the response to treatment. The simpler tests have limited value in childhood as they do not give consistently reliable results in children under the age of seven or eight years. It is often useful to repeat lung function tests after giving an inhaled bronchodilator.

Pattern of respiratory function in CF

As the child grows, there is a difference in the contribution to the total resistance to air flow produced by the smaller and larger airways. In young children, the resistance produced by the smaller airways may be as much as 50 per cent of the total, whereas in older children and adults, this forms a smaller percentage and the contribution made by the larger airways is more marked.

Impairment of respiratory function follows a typical pattern. In the early stages, *obstruction of the small airways occurs,* as a result of mucus secretion and infection. Gas exchange in the affected areas is impaired, with shunting of deoxygenated blood into the arterial system. Involvement of the *large airways* comes later. In some CF patients airways obstruction is further increased by broncho-constriction on exercise or in response to the inhalation of certain antigens — an asthmatic response.

The effect of disease in the small airways is to produce an increase in resistance to airflow. It is only when many small airways are involved that any significant change in total resistance will be detected. By contrast, quite mild disease of the large airways, such as that caused by an upper respiratory tract infection, may produce a detectable change in total airways resistance. The most sensitive indices of early disease in CF are tests which measure the function of small airways, e.g. closing volumes and maximum expiratory flow rates at 50 per cent and 25 per cent of vital capacity (as calculated from flow-volume curves, or the Vitalograph trace). Such tests are available only at specialized lung function laboratories and most are not practicable for infants and young children.

The simple lung function tests in common use are based on a forced expiration, and the result depends on the combined resistance to airflow of both large and small airways.

Simple tests of airways obstruction

Peak expiratory flow rate (PEFR) L/min This is the maximal rate at which air can be expired following a maximal inspiration. The peak flow is achieved early in a forced expiration and is usually measured with a Wright Peak Flow Meter. It depends to a considerable degree on patient co-operation and can be improved with training but once the child has mastered the knack it is simple and repeatable. Three readings are usually taken and the best of these is recorded. There is some variation between instruments and as far as possible tests should always be performed using the same one. Airways obstruction reduces PEFR.

TABLE X. Lung function values in normal children aged 7–15 years (based on Cotes JE. *Lung Function 4 Edn.* Oxford: Blackwell. 1979. Reproduced with permission)

Height (m)	Males FEV$_1$ (L)	Males FVC (L)	Males and Females PEFR (L/min)	Females FEV$_1$ (L)	Females FVC (L)
0.90			92*		
0.95			107		
1.00			124		
1.05			146		
1.10	1.06	1.30	169	1.02	1.21
1.15	1.20	1.47	192	1.15	1.36
1.20	1.35	1.65	215	1.30	1.52
1.25	1.51	1.84	238	1.45	1.69
1.30	1.68	2.05	260	1.61	1.88
1.35	1.86	2.27	283	1.79	2.07
1.40	2.06	2.51	306	1.97	2.28
1.45	2.27	2.76	329	2.17	2.49
1.50	2.50	3.02	352	2.38	2.73
1.55	2.73	3.31	374	2.61	2.97
1.60	2.99	3.61	397	2.84	3.23
1.65	3.25	3.92	419	3.09	3.50
1.70	3.53	4.25	442	3.35	3.78
1.75	3.83	4.60	465	3.63	4.08
1.80	4.14	4.97	488	3.92	4.39

* It is easier for young children to use a peak flow meter than a Vitalograph.
$\frac{FEV_1 \times 100}{FVC}$ is largely independent of age in childhood, figures being 84 per cent (males) and 88 per cent (females).

Forced expiratory volume in one second (FEV$_1$) This test measures the volume expired during the first second of a forced expiration. The instrument in widespread use in the United Kingdom is the Vitalograph. Sometimes the $FEV_{0.75}$ is used as an alternative, but it offers no advantage over the FEV_1. The results are best expressed as a percentage of the predicted normal value for the patient's height, sex and age (Table X).

Forced vital capacity (FVC) This is the total volume of air expelled during forced maximal expiration following maximal inspiration. It accounts for about three-quarters of the total lung capacity, the remaining air in the lung after full expiration being known as the residual volume. Like the FEV_1 it is measured using the Vitalograph (during the same 'blow'). The patient takes a normal inspiration and is then persuaded to continue blowing out until the flow stops, i.e. to residual volume. Clearly, with children, this requires experienced personnel. Vital capacity (VC) is measured in the same way but the expiration is unforced.

FVC increases in relation to height, sex and age (Table X). There is a later decline of both FEV_1 and FVC which begins after about 25 years (Tables XI, XII). Cystic fibrosis will eventually reduce lung capacity and thus also vital capacity and forced vital capacity.

TABLE XI. Lung function values in normal adult males, aged 20, 30 and 50 years (based on Cotes JE. *Lung Function 4 Edn.* Oxford: Blackwell. 1979. Reproduced with permission)

Height (m)	Age (Years)	FEV_1 (L)	FVC (L)	$\dfrac{FEV_1}{FVC}$ %	PEFR (L/min)
1.65	20	3.94	4.54	87	602
	30	3.60	4.32	84	577
	50	3.10	3.88	78	527
1.70	20	4.12	4.80	86	620
	30	3.81	4.58	84	594
	50	3.19	4.14	77	543
1.75	20	4.31	5.06	85	638
	30	4.00	4.84	83	612
	50	3.38	4.40	77	559
1.80	20	4.49	5.32	84	657
	30	4.18	5.10	82	629
	50	3.56	4.66	76	575

TABLE XII. Lung function values in normal adult females, aged 20, 30 and 50 years (based on Cotes JE. *Lung Function 4 Edn.* Oxford: Blackwell. 1979. Reproduced with permission)

Height (m)	Age (Years)	FEV$_1$ (L)	FVC (L)	$\dfrac{FEV_1}{FVC}$ %	PEFR (L/min)
1.55	20	2.82	3.17	89	424
	30	2.60	2.96	88	403
	50	2.16	2.54	85	361
1.60	20	2.94	3.38	87	443
	30	2.72	3.17	86	422
	50	2.28	2.75	83	379
1.65	20	3.07	3.59	85	462
	30	2.84	3.38	84	441
	50	2.41	2.96	81	398
1.70	20	3.19	3.80	84	480
	30	2.97	3.59	83	459
	50	2.53	3.17	80	417

Ratio of FEV$_1$ to FVC The FEV$_1$ is normally 70 per cent or more of the FVC and this ratio falls when there is airways obstruction.

The normal values given in Tables X, XI and XII are subject to considerable individual variation as well as any variability between individual instruments and operators. Results should only be considered abnormal if they are more than 20 per cent below predicted values. In general, for children, boys have slightly larger FEV$_1$ and FVC values than girls of the same age and stature, but PEFR is similar for both sexes (Table X). In adults, the same differences for FEV$_1$ and FVC apply but PEFR is greater for men (Tables XI, XII).

Blood gases

Measurement of PaO$_2$, PaCO$_2$ and pH in a specimen of arterial blood or 'arterialized' capillary blood is often used in the management of severely ill patients in respiratory failure. Results depend on both the underlying respiratory disease and any element of cardiac failure which may be present.

Radioisotopes

Inhalation of radioactive nitrogen (^{13}N) or xenon (^{133}Xe) and the intravenous injection of technetium labelled albumin can be used to compare ventilation and perfusion in the lungs on a regional basis. These tests are carried out rarely in CF, when localized areas of lung are considered for surgery, lavage or bronchial aspiration, and should be used in conjunction with other tests, e.g. bronchoscopy.

REFERENCES AND GENERAL READING

The sweat test

Anderson CM, Freeman M. 'Sweat test' results in normal persons of different ages compared with families with fibrocystic disease of the pancreas. *Arch Dis Childh 1960; 35:* 581–587

Bray PT, Clark GCF, Moody GJ et al. Sweat testing for cystic fibrosis: errors associated with the in situ sweat test using chloride ion selective electrodes. *Clin Chim Acta 1977; 80:* 333–338

Carter EP, Barrett AD, Heeley et al. Improved sweat test method for the diagnosis of cystic fibrosis. *Arch Dis Childh 1984; 59:* 919–922

Cogswell JJ, Risdon RA, Taylor B. Chronic suppurative lung disease in sisters mimicking cystic fibrosis. *Arch Dis Childh 1974; 49:* 520–524

Collins JE, Rolles CJ. Is the sweat test infallible in cystic fibrosis? *Acta Paediatr Scand 1985; 74:* 423–426

David TJ, Phillips BM. Overdiagnosis of cystic fibrosis. *Lancet 1982; ii:* 1204–1205

Davis PB, Hubbard VS, di Sant'Agnese PA. Low sweat electrolytes in a patient with cystic fibrosis. *Am J Med 1980; 69:* 643–645

Denning CR, Huang NN, Cuasay LR et al. Co-operative study comparing three methods of performing sweat tests to diagnose cystic fibrosis. *Pediatrics 1980; 66:* 752–757

di Sant'Agnese PA. The sweat defect in CF. In Warwick WJ, ed. *1000 Years of Cystic Fibrosis.* Minnesota: University of Minnesota. 1981: 35–47

di Sant'Agnese PA, Darling RC, Perera GA et al. Abnormal electrolyte composition of sweat in cystic fibrosis of the pancreas, clinical significance and relationship to the disease. *Pediatrics 1953; 12:* 549–563

Editorial. Cystic fibrosis variants – or variations? *Lancet 1978; ii:* 1032–1033

Editorial. Diagnosis of cystic fibrosis. *Lancet 1982; ii:* 1196–1197

Gibson LE. Reliability of sweat tests in diagnosis of cystic fibrosis. *J Pediatr 1972; 81:* 193–194

Gibson LE, Cooke RE. A test for concentration of electrolytes in sweat in cystic fibrosis of the pancreas utilizing pilocarpine by iontophoresis. *Pediatrics 1959; 23:* 545–549

Hardy JD, Davison SHH, Higgins MU et al. Sweat tests in the newborn period. *Arch Dis Childh 1973; 48:* 316–318

Hodson ME, Beldon I, Power R et al. Sweat tests to diagnose cystic fibrosis in adults. *Br Med J 1983; 286:* 1381–1383

Huff DS, Huang NN, Arey JB. Atypical cystic fibrosis of the pancreas with normal levels of sweat chloride and minimal pancreatic lesions. *J Pediatr 1979; 94:* 237–249

Kirk JM, Adams A, Westwood A et al. Measurement of osmolality and sodium concentration in heated cup sweat collections for the investigation of cystic fibrosis. *Ann Clin Biochem 1983; 20:* 369–373

Kopito L, Shwachman H. Ion-specific electrodes in diagnosis of cystic fibrosis. *Pediatrics 1968; 43:* 794–799

McKendrick T. Sweat sodium levels in normal subjects, in fibrocystic patients and their relatives, and in chronic bronchitic patients. *Lancet 1962; i:* 183–186

Sarsfield JK, Davies JM. Negative sweat tests and cystic fibrosis. *Arch Dis Childh 1975; 50:* 463–466

Schoni MH, Kraemer R, Bahler P et al. Early diagnosis of cystic fibrosis by means of sweat micro-osmometry. *J Pediatr 1984; 104:* 691–694

Schwarz V, Simpson NIM, Ahuja AS. Limitations of the diagnostic value of the sweat test. *Arch Dis Childh 1977; 52:* 870–874

Shwachman H, Goodchild MC, Khaw K-T et al. Incomplete expression of cystic fibrosis. *Cystic Fibrosis Club Abstracts 1966:* 2

Shwachman H, Mahmoodian A. Reappraisal of the chloride plate test as screening test for cystic fibrosis. *Arch Dis Childh 1981; 56:* 137–139

Shwachman H, Mahmoodian A, Neff RK. The sweat test: sodium and chloride values. *J Pediatr 1981; 98:* 576–578

Smalley CA, Addy DP, Anderson CM. Does that child really have cystic fibrosis? *Lancet 1978; ii:* 415–416

Stern RC, Boat TF, Abramowsky CR et al. Intermediate range sweat chloride concentration and pseudomonas bronchitis. *JAMA 1978; 239:* 2676–2680

Warwick WJ, Yeung W, Huange N et al. Evaluation of a new CF sweat test screening system: a co-operative study. In *Proceedings of 12th Annual Meeting EWGCF, Athens.* Athens: S Lennis. 1983: 269

Webster HL, Barlow WK. New approach to cystic fibrosis diagnosis by use of an improved sweat-induction/collection system and osmometry. *Clin Chem 1981; 27:* 385–387

Wilcken B, Towns SJ, Mellis CM. Diagnostic delay in cystic fibrosis: lessons from newborn screening. *Arch Dis Childh 1983; 58:* 863–866

Exocrine pancreatic insufficiency

Anderson CM, Burke V, Gracey M, eds. *Paediatric Gastroenterology 2nd Edn.* Oxford: Blackwell Scientific Publications. 1986: in preparation

Barr RG, Perman JA, Schoeller DA et al. Breath tests in pediatric gastrointestinal disorders. *Pediatrics 1978; 62:* 393–401

Barry RE, Barry R, Ene MD et al. Fluorescein dilaurate-tubeless test for pancreatic exocrine failure. *Lancet 1982; ii:* 742–744

Bergstrom K, Lundh G. Determination of trypsin in duodenal fluid as a test of pancreatic function. A methodological note. *Scand J Gastroenterol 1970; 5:* 533–536

Bonin A, Roy CC, Lasalle R et al. Faecal chymotrypsin: a reliable index of exocrine pancreatic function in children. *J Pediatr 1973; 83:* 594–600

Bravo E, Quattrucci S, Wilhelmi D et al. N-benzoyl-L-tyrosyl-PABA test value and its correlation with faecal fats in cystic fibrosis. In *Proceedings of 12th Annual Meeting EWGCF, Athens.* Athens: S Lennis. 1983: 104–108

Custance JM, Ryley HC, Robinson PG et al. Assessment of exocrine pancreatic function in cystic fibrosis. *Monogr Pediatr 1981; 14:* 161–165

Dandona P, Hodson M, Bell J et al. Serum immunoreactive trypsin concentrations in cystic fibrosis. *Lancet 1979; i:* 1032 (letter)

Dockter G, Nacu I, Kohlberger E. Determination of protease-cleaved p-amino-benzoic acid (PABA) in serum after oral administration of N-benzoyl-L-tyrosyl p-aminobenzoic acid (PABA-peptide) in children. *Eur J Pediatr 1981; 135:* 277–279

Fallstrom SP, Nygren CO, Olegard R. Plasma triglyceride increase after an oral fat load in malabsorption during early childhood. *Acta Paediatr Scand 1977; 66:* 111–116

Forrest DC, Wilcken B, Turner G. Screening for cystic fibrosis by a stool trypsin method. *Arch Dis Childh 1981; 56:* 151–153

Gillard BK, Cox KL, Pollack PA et al. Cystic fibrosis serum pancreatic amylase. Useful discriminator of exocrine function. *Am J Dis Child 1984; 138:* 577–580

Goldstein R, Blondheim O, Levy E et al. The fatty meal test: an alternative to stool fat analysis. *Am J Clin Nutr 1983; 38:* 763–767

Hadorn B, Zoppi G, Shmerling DH et al. Quantitative assessment of exocrine pancreatic function in infants and children. *J Pediatr 1968; 73:* 39–50

Hoek FJ, Sanders JTM, Tuenen A et al. In vitro and in vivo analysis of the PABA-test compared with the Lundh test-influence of intraluminal pH. *Gut 1981; 22:* 8–13

Junglee D, Penketh A, Katrak A et al. Serum pancreatic lipase activity in cystic fibrosis. *Br Med J 1983; 286:* 1693–1694

Kenny D, Cooke A, Tempany E et al. Activity of serum alpha amylases in cystic fibrosis. *Clin Chim Acta 1978; 89:* 429–433

McCollum JPK, Muller DPR, Harris JT. Test meal for assessing intraluminal phase of absorption in childhood. *Arch Dis Childh 1977; 52:* 887–889

Nousia-Arvanitakis SN, Arvanitakis C, Desai N et al. Diagnosis of exocrine pancreatic insufficiency in cystic fibrosis by the synthetic peptide N-benzoyl-L-tyrosyl-p-aminobenzoic acid. *J Pediatr 1978; 92:* 734–737

Sacher M, Kobsa A, Shmerling DH. PABA screening test for exocrine pancreatic function in infants and children. *Arch Dis Childh 1978; 53:* 639–641

Skude G, Kollberg H. Serum isoamylases in cystic fibrosis. *Acta Paediatr Scand 1976; 65:* 145–149

Taussig LM, Wolf RO, Woods RE et al. Use of serum amylase isoenzymes in evaluation of pancreatic function. *Pediatrics 1974; 54:* 229–235

Yamato C, Kinoshita K. A simple assay for measurement of urinary p-amino-benzoic acid in the oral pancreatic function test. *Analyt Biochem 1979; 98:* 13–17

van de Kamer JH, Huinick H ten Bokkel, Weyers HA. Rapid method for the determination of fat in faeces. *J Biol Chem 1949; 177:* 347–355

Neonatal screening

Antonowicz I, Ishida S, Shwachman H. Screening for cystic fibrosis. *Lancet 1976; i:* 746–747

Berry HK, Kellogg FW, Lichstein SR. Elevated meconium lactase activity. *Am J Dis Child 1980; 134:* 930–934

Borgstrom A, Sveger T, Lindberg T. Immunoreactive trypsin screening for cystic fibrosis. *Acta Paed Scand 1982; 71:* 621–624

Cassio A, Bernardi S, Piazzi M et al. Neonatal screening for cystic fibrosis by dried blood spot trypsin assay. *Acta Paediatr Scand 1984; 73:* 554–558

Committee Report. Neonatal screening for cystic fibrosis: position paper. *Pediatrics 1983; 72:* 741–744

Crossley JR, Elliott RB, Smith PA. Dried blood spot screening for cystic fibrosis in the newborn. *Lancet 1979; i:* 472–474

Dankert-Roelse JE, te Meerman GJ, ten Kate LP et al. Screening versus non-screening for cystic fibrosis. *Proceedings of 12th Annual Meeting EWGCF, Athens.* Athens: S Lennis. 1983: 164–168

Dodge JA, Ryley HC. Screening for cystic fibrosis. *Arch Dis Childh 1982; 57:* 774–780

Duhamel JF, Travert G, Delmas P et al. Special features of the time related evolution of IRT blood levels, in six out of seven newborns with cystic fibrosis complicated by meconium ileus. In Lawson, D, ed. *Horizons, Proceedings of the 9th International CF Congress, Brighton, England.* Chichester: John Wiley and Sons. 1984: 208

Editorial. Survival in cystic fibrosis. *Lancet 1984; i:* 663–664

Farrell PM. Early diagnosis of cystic fibrosis: to screen or not to screen – an important question. *Pediatrics 1984; 73:* 115–117

Forrest DC, Wilcken B, Turner G. Screening for cystic fibrosis by a stool trypsin method. *Arch Dis Childh 1981; 56:* 151–153

Hammond KB, Ask CG, Watts DC. Immunoreactive pancreatic lipase test for neonatal detection of cystic fibrosis. *Lancet 1984; i:* 42 (letter)

Heeley AF, Heeley ME, King DN et al. Screening for cystic fibrosis by dried blood spot trypsin assay. *Arch Dis Childh 1982; 57:* 18–21

Hellsing K, Barrljung K, Ceder O et al. Meconium screening for cystic fibrosis. *Acta Paed Scand 1982; 71:* 827–832

Holtzman NA. Routine screening for newborns for cystic fibrosis: not yet. *Pediatrics 1984; 73:* 98–99

Mastella G, Barlocco G, Braggion C et al. Long-term follow up study of CF patients diagnosed by neonatal screening or meconium ileus or symptoms. *Proceedings of 12th Annual Meeting EWGCF, Athens.* Athens: S Lennis. 1983: 169–191

Orenstein DM, Boat TF, Stern RC et al. The effect of early diagnosis and treatment in cystic fibrosis: a seven year study of 16 sibling pairs. *Am J Dis Child 1977; 131:* 973–975

Prosser R, Owen H, Bull F et al. Screening for cystic fibrosis by examination of meconium. *Arch Dis Childh 1974; 49:* 597–601

Rosenstein BJ, Langbaum TS, Metz SJ. Cystic fibrosis: diagnostic considerations. *Johns Hopkins Med J 1982; 150:* 113–120

Ryley HC, Neale LM, Brogan TD et al. Screening for cystic fibrosis in the newborn by meconium analysis. *Arch Dis Childh 1979; 54:* 92–97

Shwachman H, Antonowitz I, Mahmoodian A. Studies in meconium. An approach to screening tests to detect cystic fibrosis. *Am J Dis Child 1978; 132:* 1112–1114

Travert G, Duhamel JF. Neonatal screening for CF using IRT assay in dried blood spots: a four years' experience in Basse-Normandie. In Lawson D, ed. *Horizons, Proceedings of the 9th International CF Congress, Brighton, England.* Chichester: John Wiley and Sons. 1984: 209

Wilcken B, Brown ARD, Urwin R et al. Cystic fibrosis screening by dried blood spot trypsin assay: results in 75,000 newborn infants. *J Pediatr 1983; 102:* 383–386

Wilson JMG, Jungner G. *Principles and Practice of Screening for Disease.* Geneva: WHO. 1968

Respiratory function tests

Cotes, JE. *Lung Function. Assessment and Application in Medicine 4 Edn.* Oxford: Blackwell Scientific Publications. 1979

Cotes JE, Dabbs JM, Hall AM et al. Lung volumes, ventilatory capacity and transfer factor in healthy British boy and girl twins. *Thorax 1973; 28:* 709–715

Freedman S. Lung function tests. *Hospital Update 1981; March:* 281–293

Godfrey S, Baum JD. *Clinical Paediatric Physiology.* Oxford: Blackwell Scientific Publications. 1979

Godfrey S, Mearns M, Howlett G. Serial lung function studies in cystic fibrosis in the first 5 years of life. *Arch Dis Childh 1978; 53:* 83–85

Hiller EJ, Kirkpatrick JA, Huang NN. Radiographic determination of total lung capacity in patients with cystic fibrosis. *J Pediatr 1971; 78:* 435–440

Mearns MB. Simple tests of ventilatory capacity in children with cystic fibrosis. *Arch Dis Childh 1968; 43:* 528–539

Williams HE. In Phelan PD, Landau LI, Olinsky A, eds. *Respiratory Illness in Children 2nd Edn.* Oxford: Blackwell Scientific Publications. 1982

Chapter 11

CURRENT RESEARCH AND THE BASIC DEFECT

It is now almost 50 years since the first detailed descriptions of CF were provided by Fanconi (1936) and Andersen (1938) (see Chapter 1) and the nature of the basic biochemical defect is still unknown.

On clinical impression, the disease is associated with pulmonary and gastrointestinal secretions of increased stickiness. Examination of mucous secreting glands reveals distended glands, blockage of ducts leading from these glands and obstructive cellular damage distal to the blockage. In addition there are abnormalities of ion and water content of CF cells and secretions, the most notable being the increased salt content of sweat.

These observations have led to a study of the secretions themselves, in order to define a physical or chemical abnormality; to searches for humoral and other factors, which could influence ion transport and membrane permeability; and to an investigation of the systems which control secretions and ion transport. The basic defect will be responsible for an abnormal or an absent protein in affected tissues, but so far, this has not been identified. Meanwhile, with the expansion of techniques for the examination of chromosomes and gene mapping, much effort has been concentrated on a search for the *gene defect*. This is both to recognize the fundamental error and to assist with genetic counselling.

The gene defect

Although most of the clinical manifestations of CF are expressed by exocrine (surface secreting) cells, the CF gene will be found in *all* cells.

By analogy with other diseases inherited in a similar way, the CF basic defect is likely to be caused by a mutation (or structural abnormality) of a single gene, coding for a particular protein.

One approach is to identify the location (locus) of the abnormal gene on one of the 44 autosomes (chromosomes) within the nuclei of cells from the CF patient. This involves a process known as gene mapping. Association of cystic fibrosis either with abnormal genes or characteristics within large families, or with other diseases whose genetic loci are already known, would provide suitable starting points. There are many thousands of potential sites for a gene disorder, so a reliable clue of this kind could indicate which chromosome or part of a chromosome could carry the defective gene and so limit the number of studies which would be necessary. Essentially, in this procedure, the nucleotide structure of chromosome fragments from CF cells is compared with similar chromosome fragments from cells of unaffected individuals.

Studies of this nature are being actively carried out in a number of molecular biology centres throughout the world and while the exercise is a painstaking process it should lead ultimately to the identification of the abnormal sequence of DNA — this is the genetic material which is transmitted from parents to children and which carries the code or information which determines the characteristics of the offspring.

Once this identification has been made, it will be possible to find out the structure and eventually the function of the protein actually manufactured in the cell on the instructions of the DNA. Whether or not it will be possible to modify the functional effects of the protein abnormality (that is the fundamental disorder of CF) remains to be seen.

Isolation of the gene defect would provide an accurate test for antenatal diagnosis. It should also permit the recognition of CF carriers (heterozygotes) and so assist with genetic counselling.

Prenatal screening and heterozygote detection

A test already exists for prenatal screening (see page 8) but while this is an undoubted step forward, it is based on a secondary manifestation in the disease and not on the primary gene defect. It is also applicable only to parents who are known CF carriers.

Even now (1985), without knowledge of the primary defect, there is evidence for the existence of a 'CF protein' or 'CF marker' which is found in greater amounts in the blood of CF patients than in their obligate heterozygote parents (Wilson, Arnaud and Fudenberg, 1978; Brock, 1984). Antisera have been raised (Manson and Brock, 1980) and the system has been applied with some success to a limited number of CF patients and carriers (Bullock et al, 1982). A combination of the known statistical risks of being a CF carrier and the presence or other-wise of this protein has been employed to provide more accurate genetic counselling for couples at risk (Super and Swindlehurst, 1984).

A number of other tests have also been put forward to permit the detection of the CF carrier. However at the moment, all these tests, for both antenatal diagnosis and heterozygote detection, represent compromises and will be replaced as soon as the gene defect is identi-fied. Meanwhile, a great deal of research has been conducted, and is still continuing, to find out more about CF tissues and secretions.

Mucous secretions

Cystic fibrosis pulmonary secretions are difficult to obtain in the uninfected state. Nevertheless, considerable work has been done on these and on other mucous secretions which show that there is a change in the carbohydrate composition (Alhadeff, 1978). It is unclear, how-ever, whether this is of functional significance.

Despite the clinical impression that CF sputum is sticky, actual measurements have shown that CF sputum is no more viscous than sputum, comparably infected, from patients with bronchiectasis (Feather and Russell, 1970; King, 1981). On the other hand, CF duodenal fluid is generally slow-moving and viscous (Lorin, Denning and Mandel, 1972). It is possible that this increased viscosity is due entirely to a reduced water content (Johansen, Anderson and Hadorn, 1968; Kopelman et al, 1985).

Calcium metabolism

It has been known for some time that many CF exocrine secretions have a raised calcium concentration (Chernick, Barbero and Parkins, 1961; Gugler et al, 1967; Blomfield, Warton and Brown, 1973). More recently, much effort has been directed to the investigation of whether there is an abnormality in intracellular calcium in CF cells, but although increases have been found in certain cells, no overall picture has emerged (Katz, Schoni and Bridges, 1984; Case, 1984; Mangos and Boyd, 1984).

These studies are important because calcium exerts a controlling influence on many of the activities of the cell. Interactions may occur not only with the secretions themselves, producing altered characteristics, but with the transport of sodium and other ions and water across cell membranes (Boat and Dearborn, 1984).

Cystic fibrosis 'factors'

Abnormalities of protein and calcium content in CF exocrine secretions could be caused by a component(s) of CF serum.

CF factors, which affect the function of isolated tissues, have been recognized, although not finally characterized, since the first descriptions by Spock et al (1967) of a factor in CF serum which disorganized the beat of animal ciliated epithelium (ciliary dyskinesia) and by Mangos, McSherry and Benke (1967) of a factor in both CF sweat and CF saliva, which impaired the absorption of sodium across the sweat gland duct, so producing the increased sodium content of CF sweat.

CF serum also causes the release of mucins from exocrine gland cells (using rat submandibular cells as the model, Fleming and Sturgess, 1981; McPherson, Dodge and Goodchild, 1983) and this is in keeping with further observations on ciliary dyskinesia, when CF serum has been seen to induce a swelling of local goblet (secretory) cells, with discharge of mucus and disturbance of the adjacent cilia (Czegledy-Nagi and Sturgess, 1976; Bogart et al, 1978). The subject of serum factors has been reviewed extensively by Wilson (1983) who concluded that they are synthesized by leucocytes.

There is still no agreement on whether these factors are specific to CF, whether they are abnormal proteins or normal proteins present in excess, or how they relate to the CF protein which has been separated by isoelectric focusing techniques and used in genetic counselling (see above).

Doubt has been cast on the role of CF factors by the observation that CF nasal epithelial cells, transplanted, retained their abnormal chloride ion permeability (Yankaskas et al, 1985 and see below). Only when these factors have been fully characterized will it be possible to assess their true importance.

Electrolyte transport

Cystic fibrosis secretions are mainly of two kinds: watery, with raised electrolytes, as in sweat and saliva; concentrated, with a high protein and calcium and diminished response, by volume and bicarbonate production, to the effects of intravenous secretin, as in duodenal fluid (Johansen, Anderson and Hadorn, 1968).

Until recently, the raised electrolytes in CF sweat and saliva have been considered to be due primarily to an inhibition of the reabsorption of *sodium* across the gland ducts. The demonstration that it is the *chloride* ion which is primarily involved, with a decrease of chloride ion permeability, is an important advance (Quinton and Bijman, 1983).

This defect in the passage of the chloride ion has been found not only in sweat glands but also in respiratory epithelium (Knowles, Gatzy and Boucher, 1983; Knowles et al, 1983) and even across the placental membranes derived from a CF baby (Davis, Shennan and Boyd, 1985). The observation that placental (i.e. fetal) tissue is involved makes it extremely unlikely that the chloride transport abnormality is an acquired, secondary phenomenon. It may be that the same abnormality of chloride transport is present also across the pancreatic ducts. Reduced exit of chloride ions could be associated with a reduced entry of bicarbonate and a final secretion which is more acidic than normal (Quinton, 1984).

If this defect in chloride transport is indeed present in all affected CF tissues, a single abnormality could explain the widespread manifestations of the disease as they affect sweat secretion, lung and pancreatic function.

The reason for this difference in electrolyte transport is not known. Transport of sodium is controlled by an active process requiring energy. Chloride transport, on the other hand, appears to be through specific channels or pores which are lined by proteins attached to structural fats (Mead, 1984). An abnormality in either the protein or the fat component could be responsible.

The autonomic nervous system

Secretory activity of exocrine glands is under the control of the autonomic nervous system. Most glands are induced to secrete mainly by the parasympathetic system, but the sweat glands are innervated by the cholinergic nerves of the 'anomalous' sympathetic system. Roberts (1959) suggested that all the various manifestations of the disease could be explained by some abnormality at the neuroglandular junctions.

Although this may be too simple an approach, the principle has not been dismissed. Evidence has accumulated that autonomic nervous system responses are slightly different in CF patients (Davis, Shelhamer and Kaliner, 1980). In the laboratory, recent studies on white blood cells (Davis et al, 1983), respiratory epithelium (Knowles, Gatzy and Boucher, 1983), sweat glands (Sato and Sato, 1984; Harper and Quinton, 1984) and acinar cells from salivary glands (Mangos, 1981; McPherson et al, 1985) all indicate that there is a defect in response to beta-adrenergic stimulation in CF cells.

The significance of this altered adrenergic function in relation to other findings in CF remains to be elucidated.

Animal models

Cystic fibrosis has not been found in the animal kingdom. Rats treated with isoproterenol and reserpine, over a period of time, produce glandular enlargement and some electrolyte changes which are similar to those of cystic fibrosis. However, the rat (or any other animal) is not generally accepted as a valid model and results must be interpreted with caution.

Clinical aspects

Reference has been made earlier in this book to the importance of maintaining the quality of life by treating the secondary and tertiary manifestations of CF. A great deal of research is being directed towards finding better methods of nutrition, more effective pancreatic enzymes, better physiotherapy techniques and more powerful antibiotics.

Of particular interest and relevance to the patient is research into the treatment of pulmonary infection. Specifically, we need to know why *Pseudomonas aeruginosa* has a predilection to infect CF lungs, and why the organism undergoes the characteristic mucoid change when in the CF environment. It is entirely possible that the answers to questions like these would shed important light on the nature of the basic defect. Clearly, basic and applied research must go hand in hand if the enigma of this disease is to be solved.

REFERENCES AND GENERAL READING

Gene defect and applied genetics

Brock DJH. Prenatal screening and heterozygote detection. In Lawson D, ed. *Cystic Fibrosis: Horizons. Proceedings of the 9th International CF Congress, Brighton, England.* Chichester: John Wiley & Sons. 1984: 1–12

Brock DJH, Bedgood D, Barron L et al. Prospective prenatal diagnosis of cystic fibrosis. *Lancet 1985; i:* 1175–1178

Brock DJH, Heywood C, Super M. Controlled trial of serum isoelectric focusing in the detection of the cystic fibrosis gene. *Hum Genet 1982; 60:* 30–31

Bullock S, Hayward C, Manson J et al. Quantitative immunoassays for diagnosis and carrier detection in cystic fibrosis. *Clin Genet 1982; 21:* 336–341

Ceder O, Hosli P, Vogt E et al. Diagnosis of cystic fibrosis homozygotes and heterozygotes from plasma and fibroblast cultures. A three generation family study. *Clin Genet 1983; 23:* 298–303

Davies KE. The application of DNA recombinant technology to the analysis of the human genome and genetic disease. *Hum Genet 1981; 58:* 351–357

Jamieson A, Mackinlay E, Aitken DA et al. Quantitative variation in cystic fibrosis-associated proteins in cystic fibrosis patients, carriers and controls. *Hum Genet 1985; 70:* 168–171

Katznelson D, Blau H, Sack J. Detection of cystic fibrosis genotypes. *Lancet 1983; ii:* 622 (letter)

Lieberman J, Kaneshiro W. Identification of CF heterozygotes by a lectin-like factor and cofactor in serum utilizing S-300 gel filtration. In Lawson D, ed. *Cystic Fibrosis: Horizons. Proceedings of the 9th International CF Congress, Brighton, England.* Chichester: John Wiley & Sons. 1984: 13

Manson JC, Brock DJH. Development of a quantitative immunoassay for the cystic fibrosis gene. *Lancet 1980; i:* 330–331

Nevin GB, Nevin NC, Redmond AO et al. Detection of cystic fibrosis homozygotes and heterozygotes by serum isoelectric focusing. *Hum Genet 1981; 56:* 387–389

Super M, Swindlehurst C. Isoelectric focusing of serum in genetic counselling of families with cystic fibrosis. *Am J Med Gen 1984; 18:* 449–453

Williamson R, Casey G, Humphries S et al. Molecular genetics – basic principles and techniques. In Saunders KB, ed. *Advanced Medicine 19.* London: Pitman. 1983: 196–201

Williamson R, Gilliam C, Blaxter M et al. Gene cloning – a tool to find the basic defect in cystic fibrosis? In Lawson D, ed. *Cystic Fibrosis: Horizons. Proceedings of the 9th International CF Congress, Brighton, England.* Chichester: John Wiley & Sons. 1984: 139–153

Wilson GB, Arnaud P, Fudenberg HH. Improved method for the detection of cystic fibrosis protein in the serum using LKB multiphor electrofocusing apparatus. *Pediatr Res 1978; 12:* 801–804

Mucous secretions and viscosity

Alhadeff JA. Glycoproteins and cystic fibrosis: a review. *Clin Genet 1978; 14:* 189–201

Boat TF, Cheng PW. Glycoproteins. In Lloyd-Still JD, ed. *Cystic Fibrosis.* Boston: John Wright. 1983: 53–69

Brogan TD, Ryley HC, Neale L et al. Soluble proteins of bronchopulmonary secretions from patients with cystic fibrosis, asthma and bronchitis. *Thorax 1975; 30:* 72–79

Feather EA, Russell G. Sputum viscosity and pulmonary function in cystic fibrosis. *Arch Dis Childh 1970; 45:* 807–808

Johansen PG, Anderson CM, Hadorn B. Cystic fibrosis of the pancreas: a generalized disturbance of water and electrolyte movement in exocrine tissue. *Lancet 1968; i:* 455–460

King M. Is cystic fibrosis mucus abnormal? *Pediatr Res 1981; 15:* 120–122

Kopelman H, Durie P, Gaskin K et al. Pancreatic fluid secretion and protein hyperconcentration in cystic fibrosis. *N Engl J Med 1985; 312:* 329–334

Kopito LE, Kosasky HJ, Shwachman H. Water and electrolytes in cervical mucus from patients with cystic fibrosis. *Fert Steril 1973; 24:* 512–520

Lorin MI, Denning CR, Mandel ID. Viscosity of exocrine secretions in cystic fibrosis: sweat, duodenal fluid and submaxillary saliva. *Biorheology 1972; 9:* 27–32

Calcium metabolism

Blomfield J, Warton KL, Brown JM. Flow rate and inorganic components of submandibular saliva in cystic fibrosis. *Arch Dis Childh 1973; 48:* 267–274

Case RM. Ca^{2+} stimulus-secretion coupling and cystic fibrosis. In Lawson D, ed. *Cystic Fibrosis: Horizons. Proceedings of the 9th International Congress on Cystic Fibrosis, Brighton, England.* Chichester: John Wiley & Sons. 1984: 53–67

Chernick WS, Barbero GJ, Parkins FM. Studies on submaxillary saliva in cystic fibrosis. *J Pediatr 1961; 59:* 890–898

Forstner JF, Forstner GG. Effects of calcium on intestinal mucin: implications for cystic fibrosis. *Pediatr Res 1976; 10:* 609–613

Gibson LE, Matthews WJ, Minihan PT et al. Relating mucus, calcium, and sweat in a new concept of cystic fibrosis. *Pediatrics 1971; 48:* 695–710

Gugler E, Pallavicini JC, Swerdlow H et al. Role of calcium in submaxillary saliva of patients with cystic fibrosis. *J Pediatr 1967; 71:* 585–588

Katz S, Schoni MH, Bridges MA. The calcium hypothesis of cystic fibrosis. *Cell Calcium 1984; 5:* 421–440

Sutcliffe CH, Style PP, Schwarz V. Biochemical studies of sweat excretion in cystic fibrosis. *Proc R Soc Med 1968; 61:* 297–300

von Ruecker AA, Bertele R, Harms HK. Calcium metabolism and cystic fibrosis: mitochondrial abnormalities suggest a modification of the mitochondrial membrane. *Pediatr Res 1984; 18:* 594–599

Cystic fibrosis 'factors'

Bijman J, Quinton PM. Apparent absence of cystic fibrosis sweat factor on ion-selective and transport properties of the perfused human sweat duct. *Pediatr Res 1984; 18:* 1292–1296

Boat TF, Polony I, Cheng PW. Mucin release from rabbit tracheal epithelium in response to sera from normal and cystic fibrosis subjects. *Pediatr Res 1982; 16:* 792–797

Bogart BI, Conod EJ, Gaerlan PF et al. Biological activities of cystic fibrosis serum II. Ultrastructural aspects of the effect of cystic fibrosis sera and calcium ionophore A23187 on rabbit tracheal explants. *Pediatr Res 1978; 14:* 1173–1179

Bowman BH, Barnett DR, Carson SD et al. Studies of cystic fibrosis utilizing mucociliary activity in oyster gills. *Fed Proc 1980; 39:* 3195–3200

Conover JH, Conod EJ. The influence of cystic fibrosis serum and calcium on secretion in the rabbit tracheal mucociliary apparatus. *Biochem Biophys Res Commun 1978; 83:* 1595–1601

Czegledy-Nagy E, Sturgess JM. Cystic fibrosis: effects of serum factors on mucus secretion. *Lab Invest 1976; 35:* 585–595

Danes BS. Association of cystic fibrosis factor to metachromasia of the cultured cystic fibrosis fibroblast. *Lancet 1973; ii:* 765–767

Fleming N, Sturgess JM. Stimulation of glycoprotein secretion in dispersed rat submandibular gland acini by cystic fibrosis serum. *Experientia 1981; 37:* 139–141

Kaiser D, Drack E, Rossi E. Inhibition of net sodium transport in single human sweat glands by sweat of patients with cystic fibrosis of the pancreas. *Pediatr Res 1971; 5:* 167–172

Mangos JA, McSherry NR, Benke PJ. A sodium transport inhibitory factor in the saliva of patients with cystic fibrosis of the pancreas. *Pediatr Res 1967; 1:* 436–442

McPherson MA, Dodge JA, Goodchild MC. Cystic fibrosis serum stimulates mucin secretion but not calcium efflux from rat submandibular acini. *Clin Chim Acta 1983; 135:* 181–188

Morrissey SM, Mehta JG. Effect of cystic fibrosis and non-cystic fibrosis plasma on the movement and retention of $^{45}Ca^{2+}$ and $^{35}SO_4^{2-}$ in guinea-pig stomach and small intestine. *Gut 1981; 22:* 788–792

Spock A, Heick HMC, Cress H et al. Abnormal serum factor in patients with cystic fibrosis of the pancreas. *Pediatr Res 1967; 1:* 173–177

Wilson GB. Ciliary dyskinesia factors produced by leucocytes. In *Lymphokines, 8.* New York: Academic Press. 1983: 323–371

Wilson GB, Fudenberg HH. Ciliary dyskinesia factors in cystic fibrosis and asthma. *Nature 1977; 266:* 463–464

Yankaskas JR, Knowles MR, Gatzy JT et al. Persistence of abnormal chloride ion permeability in cystic fibrosis nasal epithelial cells in heterologous culture. *Lancet 1985; i:* 954–956

Electrolyte transport

Anderson CM. Hypothesis revisited: cystic fibrosis: a disturbance of water and electrolyte movement in exocrine secretory tissue associated with altered prostaglandin (PGE_2) metabolism? *J Pediatr Gastroenterol Nutr 1984; 3:* 15–22

Berg V, Kusoffsky E, Strandvik B. Renal function in cystic fibrosis with special reference to renal sodium handling. *Acta Paediatr Scand 1982; 71:* 833–838

Boucher RC, Ross DW, Knowles MR et al. Cl⁻ permeabilities in red blood cells and peripheral blood lymphocytes from cystic fibrosis and control subjects. *Pediatr Res 1984; 18:* 1336–1339

Davis B, Shennan DB, Boyd CAR. Chloride transport in cystic fibrosis placenta. *Lancet 1985; i:* 392–393 (letter)

Gaskin K, Durie P, Corey M et al. Evidence for a primary defect of pancreatic HCO^{-3} secretion in cystic fibrosis. *Pediatr Res 1982; 16:* 554–557

Knowles MR, Gatzy JT, Boucher RC. Relative ion permeability of normal and cystic fibrosis nasal epithelium. *J Clin Invest 1983; 71:* 1410–1417

Knowles MR, Gatzy JT, Boucher RC. Nasal transepithelial potential difference and chloride permeability in normal, cystic fibrosis and disease control subjects. In Lawson D, ed. *Cystic Fibrosis: Horizons. Proceedings of the 9th International Congress on CF, Brighton, England.* Chichester: John Wiley & Sons. 1984: 419

Knowles MR, Stutts MJ, Spock A et al. Abnormal ion permeability through cystic fibrosis respiratory epithelium. *Science 1983; 221:* 1067–1070

Mead JF. The non-eicosanoid functions of the essential fatty acids. *J Lipid Res 1984; 25:* 1517–1521

Quinton PM, Bijman J. Higher bioelectric potentials due to decreased chloride absorption in the sweat glands of patients with cystic fibrosis. *N Engl J Med 1983; 308:* 1185–1189

Widdicombe JH, Welsh MJ. Cystic fibrosis (CF) alters the electrical properties of monolayers cultured from cells of human tracheal mucosa. *Proc Nat Acad Sci 1985:* in press

Autonomic nervous system

Chernick WS, Barbero GJ, Parkins FM. Studies on submaxillary saliva in cystic fibrosis. *J Pediatr 1961; 59:* 890–898

Davis PB, Braunstein M, Jay C. Decreased adenosine 3′:5′-monophosphate response to isoproterenol in cystic fibrosis leukocytes. *Pediatr Res 1978; 12:* 703–707

Davis PB, Dieckman L, Boat TF et al. Beta-adrenergic receptors in lymphocytes and granulocytes from patients with cystic fibrosis. *J Clin Invest 1983; 71:* 1787–1795

Davis PB, Laundon SC. Adenylate cyclase in leucocytes from patients with cystic fibrosis. *J Lab Clin Med 1980; 96:* 75–84

Davis PB, Shelhamer J, Kaliner M. Abnormal adrenergic and cholinergic sensitivity in cystic fibrosis. *N Engl J Med 1980; 302:* 1453–1456

Gnegy ME, Erickson RP, Markovac J. Increased calmodulin in cultured skin fibroblasts from patients with cystic fibrosis. *Biochem Med 1981; 26:* 294–298

Harper S, Quinton PM. Adrenergic and cholinergic stimulation of CF sweat glands. In Lawson D, ed. *Cystic Fibrosis: Horizons. Proceedings of the 9th International CF Congress, Brighton, England.* Chichester: John Wiley & Sons. 1984: 178

Mangos JA. Isolated parotid acinar cells from patients with cystic fibrosis. Functional characterization. *J Dent Res 1981; 60:* 797–804

McPherson MA, Dormer RL, Dodge JA et al. Adrenergic secretory responses of submandibular tissues from control subjects and cystic fibrosis patients. *Clin Chim Acta 1985; 148:* 229–237

Roberts GBS. Fundamental defect in fibrocystic disease of the pancreas. *Lancet 1959; ii:* 964—965
Sato K, Sato F. Defective beta-adrenergic response of cystic fibrosis sweat glands in vivo and in vitro. *J Clin Invest 1984; 73:* 1763—1771

Animal models

Lebenthal E, Lee PC. Editorial. Animal models for pancreatic insufficiency in cystic fibrosis. *J Pediatr Gastroenterol Nutr 1982; 1:* 9—11
Martinez JR, Bylund DB, Mawhinney T et al. The chronically reserpinized rat as a model for cystic fibrosis: alterations in the mucus-secreting sublingual gland. *Pediatr Res 1983; 17:* 523—528
Pivetta OH, Green EL. Exocrine pancreatic insufficiency a new recessive mutation in mice. *J Hered 1973; 64:* 301—302
Pivetta OH, Sordelli DO, Labal ML. Pulmonary clearance of Staphylococcus aureus in mutant mice and some hereditary alterations resembling cystic fibrosis. *Pediatr Res 1977; 11:* 1133—1136

Clinical aspects, pseudomonas infection

Boyd RL, Mangos JA, Ramphal R. Animal model for colonization of airways by Pseudomonas aeruginosa. In Adam G, Valassi-Adam H, eds. *Proceedings of 12th Annual Meeting EWGCF, Athens, Greece.* Athens: S Lennis. 1983: 214—220
Granstrom M, Ericsson A, Strandvik B et al. Relation between antibody response to Pseudomonas aeruginosa exoproteins and colonization/infection in patients with cystic fibrosis. *Acta Paediatr Scand 1984; 73:* 772—777
Sherbrock-Cox V, Russell NJ, Gacesa P. The purification and chemical characterisation of the alginate present in extracellular material produced by mucoid strains of Pseudomonas aeruginosa. *Carbohydr Res 1984; 135:* 147—154
Wheeler WB, Williams M, Matthews WJ et al. Progression of cystic fibrosis lung disease as a function of serum immunoglobulin G levels: a 5-year longitudinal study. *J Pediatr 1984; 104:* 695—699

Reviews

Boat TF, Dearborn DG. Etiology and pathogenesis. In Taussig LM, ed. *Cystic Fibrosis.* New York: Thieme-Stratton. 1984: 25—84
Ceder O. Cystic fibrosis. In vitro and in vivo studies on the biochemical background to the pathogenesis. *Acta Paed Scand 1983:* suppl 309
Davis PB, di Sant'Agnese PA. A review. Cystic fibrosis at forty — quo vadis? *Pediat Res 1980; 14:* 83—87
di Sant'Agnese PA, Davis PB. Research in cystic fibrosis. *N Engl J Med 1976; 295:* 481—485, 534—541, 597—602
di Sant'Agnese PA, Talamo RC. Pathogenesis and pathophysiology of cystic fibrosis of the pancreas: fibrocystic disease of the pancreas (mucoviscidosis). *N Engl J Med 1967; 277:* 1287—1295, 1343—1352, 1399—1408

Mangos JA, Boyd RL. Characteristics of the CF cell. In Lawson D, ed. *Cystic Fibrosis: Horizons. Proceedings of the 9th International CF Congress, Brighton, England.* Chichester: John Wiley & Sons. 1984: 29–50

Quinton PM. Exocrine glands. In Taussig LM, ed. *Cystic Fibrosis.* New York: Thieme-Stratton. 1984: 338–375

Roussel P, Lamblin G. Trends in basic research on cystic fibrosis. In Adam G, Valessi-Adam H, eds. *Proceedings of the 12th Annual Meeting EWGCF, Athens, Greece.* Athens: S Lennis. 1983: 134–147

Sturgess JM, ed. *Perspectives in Cystic Fibrosis. Proceedings of the 8th International CF Congress, Toronto, Canada.* 1980: 3–121

Talamo RC, Rosenstein BJ, Berninger RW. Cystic fibrosis. In Stanbury JB, Wyngaarden JB, Fredrickson DS, Goldstein DS, Brown MS, eds. *The Metabolic Basis of Inherited Disease, 5th Edition, Chapter 87.* New York: McGraw Hill. 1983: 1889–1917

APPENDIX

THE CYSTIC FIBROSIS RESEARCH TRUST: OBJECTIVES, ACTIVITIES AND PUBLICATIONS

Address of Cystic Fibrosis Research Trust: Alexandra House, 5 Blyth Road, Bromley, Kent BR1 3RS, England. Telephone: 01-464-7211.

Executive Director: Mr Charles Spottiswoode

The Trust is a registered charity, founded in England in 1964. It is under the patronage of H.R.H. Princess Alexandra the Honourable Mrs Angus Ogilvy.

OBJECTIVES

These are threefold:

1. to finance research in order to find a complete cure for cystic fibrosis, and in the meantime to improve upon current methods of treatment;
2. to form regions, branches and groups throughout the United Kingdom, for the purpose of helping and advising parents with the everyday problems of caring for CF children;
3. to educate the public about the disease and, through wider knowledge, to help to promote earlier diagnosis.

ACTIVITIES

Through the local activities of its regions, branches and groups, and from a small number of national events the Trust raises funds continuously for CF research. The research projects it sponsors or supports are evaluated and monitored by the Trust's Research and Medical Advisory Committee.

In its first 20 years the Trust provided over £3.5 million for research projects and CF education. The Trust contributes to two international groups: the International Cystic Fibrosis (Mucoviscidosis) Association which organizes an International Scientific Congress every four years and the European Working Group for Cystic Fibrosis, which holds less formal scientific meetings annually. The lay organization of ICF(M)A meets annually just prior to the EWGCF scientific meeting.

The Trust also organizes regular meetings of CF research workers in the United Kingdom and clinical meetings for paediatricians and physicians who care for cystic fibrosis patients. Local and regional branch meetings are attended by parents and professional workers, and are usually addressed by visiting speakers sponsored by the Trust.

Requests for opinion on various matters concerning the welfare and management of CF patients are referred to the Trust from government bodies including the Department of Health and Social Security and the Department of Education and Science. These requests are referred to the Research and Medical Advisory Committee if necessary.

PUBLICATIONS AND VISUAL AIDS

Publications

The publications listed below are available from the Cystic Fibrosis Research Trust.

Professional

CFB/1   Proceedings of the 5th International Cystic Fibrosis Conference, Cambridge, England 1969
CFB/2   Cystic Fibrosis — Proceedings of Ciba Foundation Study Group No. 32. Published 1968
CFB/6   Low Fat Diet Cookery Book by Mary Wrigley
CFB/7   Cystic Fibrosis: Horizons. Ed. D Lawson. Proceedings of the 9th International Cystic Fibrosis Congress, Brighton, England, 1984

General

CF/1   Cystic Fibrosis by David Lawson MD, FRCP
CF/2   The Physical Treatment of Cystic Fibrosis by Diana Gaskell, MCSP and Barbara Webber, MCSP

CF/3 Living with Cystic Fibrosis. A guide for the young adult
CF/4 School teachers' leaflet
CFL/1 The Genetics of Cystic Fibrosis by C O Carter, DM, FRCP
CFL/2 CF and the Teenager by John Batten, MD, FRCP
CFL/3 Immunising the CF Child by W C Marshall, MD, PhD, FRACP, DCH
CFL/4 Cystic Fibrosis and the Social Worker by Ella MacDonald, AIMSW
CFL/5 School Problems of Children with Cystic Fibrosis by Esther E Simpson, MD
CFL/6 Diets for Children with Cystic Fibrosis by Dorothy E M Francis, SRD
CFL/7 Your CF Child at School by Heather Harston
CFL/8 Attendance Allowance (1985) by Barbara Bentley
CFL/9 Towards More Efficient Physiotherapy by Barbara Webber, MCSP
CFL/11 Research leaflet (listing current projects)
CFL/12 CF: Know the Facts: Questions and Answers

Problem? Who can help with what

To conquer Cystic Fibrosis. The first twenty years

Cystic Fibrosis News. Quarterly news from CF Trust Headquarters.

Tape/slide programme

Professional

Cystic Fibrosis –- a clinico-pathological review of cystic fibrosis for clinical students, produced by Dr R Marshall, Department of Medical Illustration, University Hospital of Wales.

Films

General

Towards a Better Future – 28 minutes. Free loan.

Living with Cystic Fibrosis – 25 minutes. Free loan. Financed by a generous grant from Tesco Stores Ltd, this film outlines the nature and effects of CF and its treatment by drugs and physiotherapy.

PROMOTIONAL MATERIAL

A wide range of promotional material including publicity and appeal posters, leaflets, car stickers and stationery, collecting aids and carnival items for resale, is available from the Trust free of charge to fundraising organizations. Full details are available on request. At Christmas time, the Trust supplies for sale Christmas cards and gift selections.

ASSOCIATION OF CYSTIC FIBROSIS ADULTS (UK)

This Association was formed in 1983. The aims and objectives are:

1. to help the CF adult to lead as full and independent a life as possible;

2. to promote the exchange of information;

3. to act as a forum for improving the management of problems encountered by CF adults, both medical and otherwise;

4. to provide encouragement for all those with CF and CF families;

5. to assist wherever possible the efforts of the CF Trust.

Interested individuals should write to:

Ann Wren, Honorary Secretary,
Association of Cystic Fibrosis Adults (UK),
288 New Road,
Ferndown,
Dorset BH22 8EP
Telephone: 0202-872405

Heidi Karlen, Honorary Secretary,
Association of Cystic Fibrosis Adults (International),
Waldstatterstrasse 6,
CH-3014 Berne,
Switzerland
Telephone: 0041-31565408

Publications

Proceedings of the 2nd International CF Adults Conference, Brighton, June 1985. Available from CF Trust Headquarters.

A regular Newsletter is also published.

INTERNATIONAL CYSTIC FIBROSIS ORGANIZATIONS

International Cystic Fibrosis Association	3567 East 49th Street, Cleveland, Ohio 44105, USA
Asociacion Argentina de Lucha contra la Enfermedad Fibroquistica del Pancreas — FIPAN	Combate de los Pozos 2193, 1245 Buenos Aires, Argentina
Australian Cystic Fibrosis Association	PO Box 225, Paddington, Queensland 4064, Australia
Osterreich Gesellschaft fur Zystische Fibrose	Universitat Kinderklinik Wien, Wahringer Gurtel 74—76, A-1097 Wien, Austria
Association Belge de Lutte Contre La Mucoviscidose	Place Georges Brugmann 29, B 1060 Brussels, Belgium
Associacão Brasileira de Assistencia a Muscoviscidose	Av Rui Barbosa 716, Botafogo, Rio de Janeiro, Brazil
Canadian Cystic Fibrosis Foundation	Suite 204, 586 Erlington Avenue East, Toronto, Ontario, Canada M4P 1P2
Comision Cubana de Fibrosis Quistica	Hospital Pediatrico Pedro Borras, Servicio de Enfermedades Respiratorias, F entre 27y29, Vedado, Habana 4, Provincia: Habana-Cuidad, Cuba
Czech Pediatric Society Committee for Cystic Fibrosis	V uvalu 84, 150 06 Prague 5, Motol, Czechoslovakia
Landsforeninger Til Bekampulse At Cystisk Fibrose	Hyrdebakken 246, DK-8800 Viborg, Denmark

Association of Pulmonary Diseases	Pohjoinen Hesperiankatu 15a, 00260 Helsinki 26, Finland
Association Francaise de Lutte contre la mucoviscidose	66 Boulevard Saint-Michel, 75006 Paris, France
Arbeitsgemeinschaft zur Bekampfung der Mukoviszidose	Kinderklinik der Medizinischen Akademie, Fetscherstrasse 74, DDR-8019 Dresden, German Democratic Republic
Deutsch Gesellschaft zur Bekampfung der Mucoviscidose (Cytische Fibrose) e.v.	Postfach 1810, 8500 Nurnberg, West Germany
Hellenic Cystic Fibrosis Group	Solonos 45, Athens 135, Greece
National Working Group for CF	Department of Pediatrics, Medical University School of Szeged, Koranyi Fasor 18, 6701 Szeged PO Box 471, Hungary
Cystic Fibrosis Association of Iceland	Barnaspitali Hringsins, Landspitalinn v/Baronsstig, Reykjavik, Iceland
Cystic Fibrosis Association Ireland	CF House, 24 Lower Rathmines Road, Dublin 6, Ireland
Cystic Fibrosis Foundation of Israel	PO Box 31171, Tel-Aviv, Israel
Societa Italiana di Pediatria Associazione Italiana per la Fibrosi Cistica	30026 Portogruaro, Venezia, Italy

Cystic Fibrosis Jordan	University of Jordan, PO Box 13350 Amman Jordan
Association Mexicana de Fibrosis Quistica	Ave revolucion 1389, 01040 Mexico, DF, Mexico
Nederlandse Cystic Fibrosis Stichting	Postbus 30, 3830 AA Leusden, The Netherlands
Cystic Fibrosis Association of New Zealand (Inc)	PO Box 1755, Wellington, New Zealand
Norsk Forening for Cystisk Fibrose	Nils Hansens vei 2, Oslo 6, Norway
Polish Cystic Fibrosis Association	National Research Institute of Mother and Child, 01-211 Warszawa, ul Kasprazaka 17, Poland
Southern African Cystic Fibrosis Association	PO Box 2, Isando 1600, Transvaal, Republic of South Africa
Asociacion Espanola contra la Fibrosis Quistica,	Avda S Antonio M Claret, 167, Barcelona 25, Spain
Riksforening for Cystic Fibrosis	Box 3049, 75003 Uppsala, Sweden
Swiss Cystic Fibrosis Association	Fliederweg 45, CH 3138 Uetendorf, Switzerland

Cystic Fibrosis Foundation   6000 Executive Blvd, Suite 309,
Rockville MD 20852,
USA

Cystic Fibrosis Association   Mother and Child Health Institute of
of Yugoslavia   Serbia,
8 Radoja Dakica St,
11071 Novi Beograd,
Yugoslavia

INDEX

(Figures in italics indicate pages containing illustrations or tables)